I0767148

Nature's Key to Be M.D. Free – A Guide to Alternative and Herbal Remedies
Second Edition

ISBN: 9798878088473

Cover Design by JM Eads

Contents

Second Edition Foreword:

Thank you for your interest in the second edition of Alternative Healing - The Secret of Herbs: Using Nature for Better Health! **This edition features the inclusion of 48 additional herbs and minerals that can be utilized in your journey to finding natural solutions to various conditions and on your pathway to overall healthier alternatives than pharmaceutical medications.**

Although some of the herbal substances included in this version are less common to find simply at a regular grocery store, but they can be attained through various channels such as online or at dedicated drug stores.

Please remember that the information in this book is provided for informational purposes only. It is for you to use your best judgment in determining whether or not the remedies included are right for you. If you take prescription medications for a condition, it is for you to discuss with your doctor to determine if the alternative herbs are a better fit for the problem than the medications.

Of course, remember that you must use YOUR best judgment in making the decision, as you are the person who your health affects the most. Remember when trying less common herbal substances it is important to start slow to ensure your body is suited to utilizing them.

INTRODUCTION

Many people in recent times have become aware of the fact that the Healthcare Industry is not so much concerned with keeping people healthy, but rather with the internal wheel of exchanged money that is received from them profiting off of your illness and overall pain. In the United States doctors are not educated on determining the underlying cause of issues that arise in the body, but rather how to use pharmaceuticals to provide relief of the symptoms. If you have ever seen commercials for a medication, you have probably noticed that the main duration of the commercial is spent listing side effects of the medication. The first red flag that you may be a lifelong guinea pig in a dance of pharmaceutical corruption is if instead of attempting to resolve an issue utilizing health improving tactics like increasing physical activity, modifying certain food choices or verifying you are receiving the proper level of VITAL nutrients in your diet (which is not likely as our modern food choices have been made void of nutritional value due to heavy processing and genetic modification of almost any items available in a supermarket or grocery store).

If your doctor's immediate choice is to put you on a medication, you should be aware that most medications simply mask the symptoms of the underlying issue. Thus, only providing relief if you continuously utilize them. This means that in most cases you will be taking these medications for the rest of your life and all the while it is likely they are causing damage to other systems and functions in your body that will overtime develop into the need you may end up having to take a specialty medication (for chronic conditions like psoriasis or rheumatoid arthritis) and these medications can cost over $10,000/month. Better hope you don't lose your job!

In a perfect world, we could assume that these doctors are acting in the best of faith to provide you with a better level of health. But as we have seen in recent years, this may no longer be the case due to backroom deals, pharmaceutical lobbying, and the fact that people are so obsessed with profits that the reality seems to be that they are prescribing medications based on the medication companies who provide the most rewards. So don't be surprised when you go to the doctor and receive an Ozempic notepad and a Lexapro pen, that just means they have incentive to prescribe these medications more.

With this in mind, it is no wonder people are turning to naturopathic or "natural" methods of healing the body. With the research and amazing results found from Barbara O'Neil and other individuals who spread a message of utilizing natural herbs and remedies that were used in days past, it came of no surprise to me that the results of utilizing these methods would provide healthier modes of living. I used to suffer from high cholesterol and high blood pressure. When I saw a video of Mrs. O'Neil stating that

Cayenne Pepper could be used to regulate blood pressure, I began the daily ritual of mixing 1 tsp. of cayenne pepper into water and drinking it. While yes, it is spicy and unpleasant to do, the results spoke for themselves as my blood pressure lowered with no medications. Because of this I decided to research natural remedies and provide a list of my findings so that people could utilize natural methods instead of pharmaceuticals. However, it is not recommended that you use this book to replace licensed medical advice from your doctor. Utilize your best judgement to decide if any herb or supplement listed here should replace a prescribed medication. I am not a licensed medical doctor and cannot provide health advice.

Please also remember that if you start an alternative remedy the results will likely not be immediate. It is important to be consistent with what you do as your body has to acclimate having the nutrients that it has previously been denied. It may take time, but in most cases, you will begin to notice significant changes in various areas pertaining to your health. And this is the goal of this work. To help give you a beginner's guide that you can utilize to learn more about the power of nature. Remember that in the olden days, they did not have medications and utilized various natural remedies that in most cases worked wonders without requiring you to spend large sums of money or remain on the medication for the remainder of your life.

Thank you for your interest in this work!

ALOE VERA

Aloe vera is a succulent plant species widely known for its therapeutic and medicinal properties. It's native to the Arabian Peninsula but cultivated in various regions worldwide for its numerous uses in traditional medicine, skincare, and even culinary applications.

Here are some key characteristics and uses of aloe vera:

- **Appearance:** Aloe vera plants typically have thick, fleshy, spear-like leaves that grow in a rosette pattern. The leaves contain a gel-like substance that's often used for its healing properties.

- **Gel and Latex:** Aloe vera contains two main substances—gel and latex. The gel, found in the inner leaf, is a clear, jelly-like substance that is used topically for its soothing, moisturizing, and healing properties. The latex, found just under the plant's skin, is a yellowish substance that is often used as a laxative.

- **Skin Benefits:** Aloe vera gel is widely utilized in skincare due to its hydrating, anti-inflammatory, and soothing effects. It's often applied topically to treat sunburns, minor cuts, wounds, eczema, and other skin irritations.

- **Nutritional Value:** Aloe vera contains vitamins, minerals, amino acids, and antioxidants that contribute to its health benefits. Some people also consume aloe vera juice for its potential digestive health benefits, although its consumption should be done cautiously and in moderation due to potential laxative effects from the latex component.

- **Commercial Uses:** Beyond skincare, aloe vera is an ingredient in various products such as lotions, creams, shampoos, and even beverages and dietary supplements.

- **Cultural and Historical Use:** Aloe vera has a long history of use in different cultures, dating back to ancient Egypt, where it was known as the "plant of immortality" and used for its healing properties. Throughout history, it's been used for various medicinal purposes.

HEALTH BENEFITS:

1. **Skin Health:** Aloe vera gel is widely used for its skin-soothing properties. It's applied topically to treat sunburns, minor burns, wounds, cuts, insect bites, and various skin irritations. It helps moisturize the skin, reduce inflammation, and promote healing.

2. **Moisturizing and Anti-Aging:** Due to its hydrating properties and the presence of antioxidants like vitamins C and E, aloe vera is included in many skincare products to help hydrate the skin and potentially reduce signs of aging.

3. **Wound Healing:** Aloe vera's compounds contribute to its ability to accelerate wound healing. It's believed to enhance the production of collagen, promoting faster healing of wounds, and reducing the risk of infection.

4. **Digestive Health:** Aloe vera juice is sometimes consumed for its potential benefits to the digestive system. It may aid in soothing and supporting digestive issues like acid reflux, indigestion, and irritable bowel syndrome (IBS). However, its consumption should be done cautiously and in moderation due to potential laxative effects.

5. **Anti-Inflammatory Effects:** Aloe vera contains compounds like polysaccharides and enzymes that exhibit anti-inflammatory properties, potentially providing relief for conditions such as arthritis and inflammatory skin conditions.

6. **Dental Health:** Some toothpaste and mouthwash formulations include aloe vera due to its potential for promoting dental health. It may help reduce plaque and gum inflammation.

7. **Antioxidant Properties:** Aloe vera contains various antioxidants that can help neutralize free radicals in the body, potentially reducing oxidative stress and lowering the risk of chronic diseases.

8. **Supporting the Immune System:** Some research suggests that aloe vera may have immune-boosting properties, contributing to overall immune health.

ANDROGRAPHIS

Andrographis, scientifically known as Andrographis paniculata, is an herbaceous plant native to South Asian countries such as India and Sri Lanka, as well as parts of Southeast Asia. It's commonly referred to as the "King of Bitters" due to its extremely bitter taste. This plant has been used for centuries in traditional medicine systems, particularly in Ayurveda, Traditional Chinese Medicine (TCM), and Southeast Asian herbal medicine.

- **Appearance:** It's an annual herb that typically grows to about 30–110 cm in height. It has lance-shaped leaves and small, tubular flowers that are usually white with hints of purple.

- **Active Compounds:** The herb contains various bioactive compounds, notably andrographolides, which are believed to be responsible for many of its health-promoting properties.

- **Health Benefits:** Andrographis is primarily known for its potential immune-boosting properties. It's often used to support the immune system, particularly during periods of colds, flu, and other infections. Additionally, it's believed to have anti-inflammatory and antioxidant properties.

- **Traditional Uses:** In traditional medicine, Andrographis has been used to alleviate fever, coughs, sore throat, and upper respiratory infections. It's also thought to support digestive health and exhibit hepatoprotective (liver-protecting) effects.

- **Forms of Use:** It's available in various forms such as capsules, tablets, tinctures, and teas, making it convenient for consumption.

- **Safety and Precautions:** While generally considered safe when used appropriately, high doses or prolonged use may cause gastrointestinal upset in some individuals. Pregnant or breastfeeding women and those with autoimmune conditions should consult a healthcare professional before using Andrographis supplements.

HEALTH BENEFITS:

1. **Immune Support:** It's often used to support the immune system, especially during cold and flu seasons. Andrographis is believed to help the body fight off infections and reduce the severity and duration of illnesses.

2. **Respiratory Health:** Due to its immune-boosting properties, Andrographis is used to address respiratory issues such as coughs, sore throat, bronchitis, and sinusitis. It may help alleviate symptoms and support recovery from these conditions.

3. **Anti-Inflammatory Effects:** Andrographis is known for its potential anti-inflammatory properties, which may be beneficial for conditions involving inflammation, such as arthritis or inflammatory bowel diseases.

4. **Antioxidant Activity:** Its compounds exhibit antioxidant effects, helping to combat oxidative stress in the body and potentially reducing the risk of chronic diseases associated with free radicals.

5. **Digestive Support:** Some traditional uses of Andrographis involve aiding digestive issues like indigestion, diarrhea, and stomach discomfort. It's believed to have a soothing effect on the gastrointestinal tract.

6. **Liver Health:** Andrographis is thought to support liver function and may be used in liver detoxification protocols due to its hepatoprotective properties.

7. **Antimicrobial Properties:** It's considered to have antimicrobial effects against certain bacteria and viruses, contributing to its use in fighting infections.

ARTEMISIA ANNUA

Artemisia annua, commonly known as sweet wormwood or Qinghao, is an herbaceous plant that has garnered attention for its potential medicinal properties, particularly in the realm of traditional medicine and as a source of an essential antimalarial compound.

Key characteristics of Artemisia annua include:

- **Appearance:** It's an annual herbaceous plant that typically grows up to 2 meters in height. The leaves are finely divided and silvery-green in color, giving the plant a feathery appearance.

- **Active Compound:** Artemisia annua contains a compound called artemisinin, which is known for its potent antimalarial properties. Artemisinin and its derivatives are used in combination therapies to treat malaria.

- **Medicinal Uses:** Traditionally, Artemisia annua has been used in Chinese medicine for treating fevers and various conditions associated with heat, and it was discovered to be effective against malaria in the 1968s. Its active compound, artemisinin, is crucial in current antimalarial drug treatments due to its ability to rapidly reduce the number of parasites in the bloodstream.

- **Scientific Interest:** Apart from its antimalarial properties, Artemisia annua is also being researched for its potential in treating other diseases, including cancer. Some studies suggest that artemisinin and its derivatives may have anticancer properties, though further research is needed in this area.

- **Cultivation:** Artemisia annua is grown in various parts of the world, particularly in regions with temperate climates. It's cultivated for its medicinal properties and the extraction of artemisinin for pharmaceutical purposes.

- **Caution:** While Artemisia annua and artemisinin are valuable in combating malaria, the emergence of drug-resistant malaria strains emphasizes the importance of using artemisinin-based therapies in combination with other antimalarial drugs, as recommended by healthcare professionals and global health organizations.

Health Benefits:

1. **Antimalarial Properties:** The most well-known benefit of Artemisia annua is its effectiveness against malaria. Artemisinin, the active compound derived from the plant, is a key component in artemisinin-based combination therapies (ACTs), which are highly effective in treating malaria, especially drug-resistant strains.

2. **Antioxidant Effects:** Some studies suggest that Artemisia annua and its compounds possess antioxidant properties. Antioxidants help neutralize free radicals in the body, potentially reducing oxidative stress and lowering the risk of chronic diseases.

3. **Anticancer Potential:** There's ongoing research exploring the potential of artemisinin and its derivatives in fighting cancer. Some studies have shown promising results in inhibiting the growth of certain cancer cells, though more research is needed to determine its efficacy and safety for cancer treatment.

4. **Anti-inflammatory Properties:** Artemisinin may possess anti-inflammatory effects, which could potentially be beneficial in conditions characterized by inflammation, although more research is needed in this area.

5. **Antibacterial and Antiviral Effects:** Some studies suggest that Artemisia annua extracts may exhibit antibacterial and antiviral properties, indicating potential use in combating certain infections. However, further research is required to confirm these effects and their applications.

While Artemisia annua shows promise in various health areas beyond its primary use in treating malaria, it's essential to approach its use cautiously and under medical guidance. Artemisinin-based therapies for malaria treatment should always be used as prescribed by healthcare professionals to avoid the development of drug resistance. Additionally, the use of Artemisia annua for other health purposes requires further scientific validation and should be undertaken with appropriate medical supervision.

Ashwagandha, scientifically known as Withania somnifera, is a medicinal herb deeply rooted in traditional Ayurvedic medicine. It's also referred to as Indian ginseng or winter cherry and has gained popularity for its potential health benefits and adaptogenic properties.

Key features and uses of ashwagandha include:

- **Adaptogenic Properties:** Ashwagandha is classified as an adaptogen, which means it may help the body adapt to stress by normalizing physiological functions. It's believed to support the body's ability to cope with stress, anxiety, and fatigue.

- **Traditional Uses:** In Ayurveda, ashwagandha has been used for centuries for its rejuvenating properties, promoting vitality, strength, and overall wellness. It's often used to enhance energy levels and improve stamina.

- **Forms of Use:** Ashwagandha is available in various forms, including powders, capsules, extracts, and teas, making it convenient for consumption.

HEALTH BENEFITS:

1. **Stress Reduction and Anxiety Relief:** Ashwagandha is renowned for its adaptogenic properties, which may help the body better manage stress. It's believed to regulate cortisol levels, reducing stress and anxiety and promoting a calmer state of mind.

2. **Enhanced Energy and Stamina:** Regular use of ashwagandha may contribute to increased energy levels and improved stamina. It's often used to combat fatigue and boost overall vitality.

3. **Improved Cognitive Function:** Some studies suggest that ashwagandha may support cognitive health by enhancing memory, focus, and overall brain function. It's believed to have neuroprotective effects that could benefit cognitive abilities.

4. **Potential Anti-Inflammatory Effects:** Ashwagandha is thought to possess anti-inflammatory properties, which may help reduce inflammation in the body. This could potentially alleviate symptoms in conditions related to inflammation, such as arthritis.

5. **Hormonal Balance:** It's suggested that ashwagandha may help balance hormones, particularly in individuals experiencing stress-related hormonal imbalances. It may support thyroid function and contribute to overall hormonal harmony.

6. **Immune Support:** Ashwagandha's immunomodulatory properties may assist in bolstering the immune system, potentially improving the body's ability to fight infections and illnesses.

7. **Support for Physical Performance:** Some research indicates that ashwagandha could aid in physical performance and strength, making it of interest to athletes or those looking to improve exercise endurance.

8. **Mood Enhancement:** Ashwagandha's ability to reduce stress and anxiety may positively impact mood and overall well-being. It's believed to have antidepressant effects, potentially alleviating symptoms of depression.

While ashwagandha shows promise in providing these health benefits, individual responses may vary. It's essential to use it cautiously, especially when combining it with other medications or supplements. Consulting a healthcare professional before starting any new supplement, especially if you have underlying health conditions or are pregnant or breastfeeding, is recommended.

BACOPA

Bacopa, scientifically known as Bacopa monnieri, is a perennial herb that is native to wetlands and marshy areas in India, North America, Europe, and Australia. It is commonly referred to as Brahmi in Ayurvedic medicine, not to be confused with Gotu Kola, which is also sometimes called Brahmi.

Key characteristics of Bacopa include:

- **Appearance:** Bacopa is a creeping herb with succulent leaves that are small, thick, and oblong. It often grows low to the ground and can form dense mats.

- **Traditional Use:** In traditional Ayurvedic medicine, Bacopa has been used to enhance cognitive function, improve memory, and reduce anxiety. It is considered an adaptogen, helping the body adapt to stress.

- **Active Compounds:** The plant contains various active compounds, including bacosides, which are believed to have neuroprotective and antioxidant properties.

- **Growing Conditions:** It thrives in aquatic or semi-aquatic conditions and is often found in marshy areas, along the edges of ponds, and in other waterlogged environments.

- **Supplement Form:** Bacopa supplements are available in various forms, including capsules, powders, and liquid extracts. These supplements are commonly used to support cognitive health.

HEALTH BENEFITS:

1. **Cognitive Enhancement:** Bacopa is recognized for its potential to enhance cognitive function, including improvements in memory and learning. Its active compounds, such as bacosides, are thought to play a role in supporting brain health.

2. **Adaptogenic Properties:** As an adaptogen, Bacopa may assist the body in adapting to stress and maintaining a balanced stress response. This adaptogenic quality is valued for its potential to mitigate the effects of stress on the body.

3. **Neuroprotective Effects:** The herb contains compounds that exhibit neuroprotective properties. These properties may help protect nerve cells from damage and support overall neurological health.

4. **Antioxidant Activity:** Bacopa is known to possess antioxidant properties, which can help combat oxidative stress in the body. Antioxidants play a crucial role in neutralizing free radicals, contributing to overall cellular health.

5. **Anxiolytic Effects:** Some studies suggest that Bacopa may have anxiolytic (anxiety-reducing) effects. This aspect can be beneficial for individuals looking to manage stress and anxiety levels.

6. **Anti-Inflammatory Potential:** Bacopa has been associated with anti-inflammatory effects, which may contribute to its overall health-promoting properties. Chronic inflammation is linked to various health issues, and the anti-inflammatory potential of Bacopa is considered beneficial.

7. **Cardioprotective Qualities:** Emerging research indicates that Bacopa may have cardioprotective effects, including potential benefits for cardiovascular health. This aspect adds to its overall positive impact on well-being.

BAOBAB:

Baobab refers to a group of trees belonging to the genus Adansonia, and they are known for their unique appearance and the distinctive characteristics of their fruit. There are several species of baobab trees, and they are native to various regions of Africa, Madagascar, Australia, and the Arabian Peninsula. Here are key features and aspects related to baobab:

- **Distinctive Appearance:** Baobab trees are easily recognizable due to their massive, swollen trunks, which can store water. The trunk's bulbous shape has led to the nickname "the upside-down tree." The branches of baobabs often resemble roots, giving them an unusual appearance.

- **Lifespan:** Baobab trees are known for their longevity, with some specimens believed to live for thousands of years. They are considered iconic and culturally significant in many African societies.

- **Fruit:** The fruit of the baobab tree is known as baobab fruit or monkey bread. It has a hard, woody shell and contains a powdery pulp with a tangy flavor. The pulp is rich in nutrients, including vitamin C, calcium, potassium, and antioxidants.

- **Nutritional Benefits:** Baobab fruit pulp is sought after for its nutritional benefits. It is particularly known for its high vitamin C content, which contributes to immune system support. The fruit pulp is also used for its potential antioxidant and anti-inflammatory properties.

- **Traditional Uses:** In various African cultures, different parts of the baobab tree have traditional uses. The leaves, bark, and fruit are utilized for medicinal purposes, and the tree itself often holds cultural significance.

- **Ecological Importance:** Baobab trees play a crucial role in the ecosystems where they grow. They provide habitat and sustenance for various animals, and their presence is vital for maintaining biodiversity in certain regions.

- **Adaptation to Arid Environments:** Baobab trees are well-adapted to arid and semi-arid environments. Their ability to store water in their trunks allows them to survive in regions with unpredictable rainfall.

- **Commercial Uses:** Beyond traditional and local uses, baobab products, particularly the fruit powder, have gained commercial interest. Baobab powder is sometimes used as a dietary supplement, and the fruit is incorporated into various food and beverage products.

HEALTH BENEFITS:

1. **Rich in Vitamin C:** Baobab fruit pulp is exceptionally high in vitamin C, contributing to immune system support. The abundance of this essential vitamin aids in protecting the body against infections and promoting overall immune health.

2. **Antioxidant Power:** The fruit's pulp is packed with antioxidants, which play a crucial role in neutralizing free radicals. Antioxidants help combat oxidative stress, potentially reducing the risk of chronic diseases and supporting overall well-being.

3. **Dietary Fiber Source:** Baobab is a good source of dietary fiber. Adequate fiber intake supports digestive health, helps regulate

bowel movements, and may contribute to weight management by promoting a feeling of fullness.

4. **Essential Minerals:** In addition to vitamin C, baobab contains essential minerals such as calcium, potassium, and magnesium. These minerals are vital for bone health, muscle function, and overall electrolyte balance in the body.

5. **Anti-Inflammatory Properties:** Some studies suggest that baobab may possess anti-inflammatory properties. This can be beneficial in managing inflammation, a factor associated with various chronic diseases.

6. **Hydration Support:** The ability of baobab trees to store water in their trunks is reflected in the hydrating properties of the fruit. Consuming baobab may contribute to overall hydration, supporting skin health and bodily functions.

7. **Energy Metabolism:** The presence of essential nutrients in baobab, including B-vitamins, supports energy metabolism. These vitamins play a role in converting food into energy, promoting vitality and overall metabolic health.

8. **Blood Sugar Regulation:** Some research indicates that baobab may have a positive impact on blood sugar levels. This potential benefit can be valuable in supporting individuals with diabetes or those looking to manage blood sugar levels.

9. **Heart Health:** The combination of antioxidants and essential minerals in baobab contributes to cardiovascular health. These elements may help in maintaining healthy blood pressure and reducing the risk of heart-related issues.

10. **Natural Anti-Microbial Properties:** Certain compounds in baobab may exhibit natural anti-microbial properties, contributing to immune defense against harmful microorganisms.

Incorporating baobab into a balanced diet can offer a variety of health advantages, making it a nutrient-rich and functional food choice. As with any dietary supplement, it's advisable to consult with a healthcare professional, especially for individuals with specific health concerns or conditions.

BERGAMOT

Bergamot refers to both a citrus fruit and the essential oil extracted from its peel. The fruit is a small, pear-shaped citrus that is believed to be a hybrid of lemon and bitter orange. It is primarily grown in the Calabria region of Southern Italy, although it is also cultivated in other parts of the world.

The peel of the bergamot fruit is highly fragrant and is used to produce bergamot essential oil, which is widely used in the perfume and cosmetics industries. The distinctive aroma of bergamot is citrusy, with floral and spicy undertones, making it a popular choice for adding fragrance to various products.

In addition to its aromatic uses, bergamot is also used in the culinary world. The zest or oil of bergamot is often added to flavor teas, candies, and desserts. One of the most well-known uses of bergamot in the culinary realm is Earl Grey tea, where the oil is blended with black tea to create a unique and aromatic beverage.

Bergamot oil is also known for its potential health benefits. It is believed to have calming and uplifting properties, and some people use it in aromatherapy for relaxation and stress relief. However, it's important to note that essential oils should be used with caution, and it's advisable to consult with a healthcare professional before using them for therapeutic purposes.

HEALTH BENEFITS

1. **Antioxidant Properties:** Bergamot contains compounds with antioxidant properties that may help neutralize free radicals in the body.

2. **Cholesterol Regulation:** Some studies suggest that bergamot may have a positive impact on cholesterol levels, potentially lowering LDL (bad) cholesterol and increasing HDL (good) cholesterol.

3. **Heart Health:** Due to its cholesterol-lowering effects and potential to improve blood vessel function, bergamot may contribute to cardiovascular health.

4. **Antibacterial Properties:** Bergamot oil has been investigated for its antibacterial properties, which may help combat certain types of bacteria.

5. **Anti-Inflammatory Effects:** Components in bergamot may exhibit anti-inflammatory effects, making it a potential candidate for managing inflammatory conditions.

6. **Mood Enhancement:** The aroma of bergamot is often used in aromatherapy for its calming and uplifting effects, which may contribute to improved mood and reduced stress.

7. **Digestive Aid:** Bergamot is sometimes used to help with digestive issues, as it may have mild digestive-stimulating properties.

8. **Skin Care:** Bergamot oil is used in skincare products for its potential to promote healthy skin and address issues like acne and oily skin.

9. **Antiviral Activity:** Some studies have explored the antiviral properties of bergamot, suggesting it may have activity against certain viruses.

10. **Blood Sugar Regulation:** There is some research indicating that bergamot may play a role in regulating blood sugar levels, which could be beneficial for individuals with diabetes or those at risk.

Remember, while these potential health benefits exist, individual responses can vary, and it's crucial to consult with a healthcare professional before using bergamot or its derivatives for therapeutic purposes.

Black Cohosh

Black cohosh (Actaea racemosa or Cimicifuga racemosa) is a perennial herb native to North America. It is known for its tall, feathery white flowers and has a long history of traditional use, particularly among Native American communities. The plant has been used for various medicinal purposes, and its root is the part most commonly utilized.

Key characteristics and uses of black cohosh include:

- **Botanical Features:** Black cohosh is a member of the buttercup family (Ranunculaceae) and typically grows in wooded areas. It has large, compound leaves and produces a spike of small white flowers in late spring to early summer.

- **Medicinal Uses:** Traditionally, black cohosh has been used to address various health concerns, particularly by Indigenous peoples. It gained popularity in the 19th century as a remedy for women's health issues, such as menstrual discomfort and menopausal symptoms.

- **Safety Considerations:** While black cohosh is generally considered safe for short-term use, there have been reports of liver toxicity associated with its consumption. It's crucial to use it under the guidance of a healthcare professional, especially for individuals with liver conditions.

- **Available Forms:** Black cohosh supplements are commonly available in various forms, including capsules, tablets, and liquid extracts. It is essential to follow recommended dosages and consult with a healthcare provider before using it, especially for prolonged periods.

1. **Menopausal Symptom Relief:** Black cohosh has been traditionally used to alleviate symptoms associated with menopause, including hot flashes, mood swings, and sleep disturbances.

2. **Menstrual Discomfort:** The herb has been used to address menstrual discomfort and may have potential benefits for women experiencing premenstrual symptoms.

3. **Estrogenic Effects:** Black cohosh is believed to have mild estrogenic activity, interacting with estrogen receptors and contributing to its effects on women's health.

4. **Anti-Inflammatory Properties:** Some studies suggest that black cohosh may have anti-inflammatory effects, making it potentially relevant for conditions involving inflammation.

5. **Bone Health:** There is some research indicating that black cohosh might have a positive impact on bone density, which could be beneficial for bone health.

6. **Anxiety and Mood:** Black cohosh has been explored for its potential to reduce anxiety and improve mood, though more research is needed to establish these effects conclusively.

7. **Cognitive Function:** There is some preliminary evidence suggesting that black cohosh might have cognitive benefits, but further research is required to confirm and understand these effects.

8. **Anti-Spasmotic Properties:** Black cohosh has been traditionally used as an antispasmodic agent, potentially helping to relax muscles and alleviate muscle cramps.

9. **Cardiovascular Health:** Some studies have investigated the impact of black cohosh on cardiovascular health, with indications that it may have positive effects, but more research is needed for conclusive evidence.

10. **Safety for Short-Term Use:** Black cohosh is generally considered safe for short-term use. However, it's essential to use it under the guidance of a healthcare professional, especially for individuals with pre-existing health conditions.

Remember that individual responses to herbal remedies can vary, and it's crucial to consult with a healthcare professional before using black cohosh, especially for prolonged periods or in combination with other medications.

BOSWELLIA

Boswellia is a genus of trees and shrubs known for producing resin with medicinal properties. The most well-known species is Boswellia serrata, also referred to as Indian frankincense. The resin, commonly known as frankincense, has been used for centuries in traditional medicine and religious ceremonies.

Here are key points about Boswellia:

1. **Botanical Features:** Boswellia trees are typically small to medium-sized and are native to the arid regions of the Middle East, Northern Africa, and India. The trees have papery bark and pinnate leaves.

2. **Resin (Frankincense):** The resin produced by Boswellia trees, known as frankincense, is obtained by making incisions in the bark. Once harvested, the resin can be used in its raw form or processed into essential oil.

3. **Traditional Uses:** Boswellia resin has a long history of use in traditional medicine, particularly in Ayurvedic and traditional Chinese medicine. It has been used to address various health issues, including inflammatory conditions, arthritis, and respiratory ailments.

4. **Aromatherapy:** Boswellia essential oil, derived from the resin, is used in aromatherapy for its calming and grounding effects. It is believed to have properties that promote relaxation and emotional well-being.

HEALTH BENEFITS

1. **Anti-Inflammatory Properties:** Boswellia has compounds, such as boswellic acids, that exhibit anti-inflammatory effects, potentially aiding in the management of inflammatory conditions.

2. **Joint Health Support:** Boswellia has been studied for its potential benefits in managing joint conditions like osteoarthritis and rheumatoid arthritis, providing relief from symptoms.

3. **Respiratory Support:** Traditional uses of Boswellia include respiratory support, making it beneficial for conditions such as asthma and bronchitis.

4. **Anti-Cancer Potential:** Ongoing research suggests that Boswellia may have anti-cancer properties, inhibiting the growth of certain cancer cells, though more studies are needed for conclusive evidence.

5. **Emotional Well-being:** Boswellia essential oil is used in aromatherapy for its calming and grounding effects, promoting relaxation and emotional well-being.

6. **Digestive Health:** Boswellia may have benefits for digestive health, with some traditional uses focusing on its ability to address digestive issues.

7. **Wound Healing:** Boswellia has been used traditionally for wound healing, and some studies suggest that it may have properties that support the skin's natural healing processes.

8. **Antioxidant Effects:** The resin of Boswellia contains compounds with antioxidant properties, which can help neutralize free radicals in the body.

9. **Anti-Asthmatic Properties:** Boswellia has been investigated for its potential anti-asthmatic effects, suggesting it may be beneficial for individuals with asthma.

10. **Anti-Bacterial Properties:** Some research indicates that Boswellia may possess antibacterial properties, contributing to its traditional use for various infectious conditions.

It's important to note that while Boswellia has potential health benefits, individual responses can vary. Consultation with a healthcare professional is advisable, especially if considering the use of Boswellia supplements or essential oil for therapeutic purposes.

BURDOCK ROOT:

Burdock root, scientifically known as Arctium lappa, is a plant native to Europe and Asia, although it's now grown in various parts of the world. It's a biennial herb that belongs to the daisy family and is well-known for its potential health benefits.

Here are key characteristics and uses of burdock root:

- **Appearance:** Burdock is a robust plant with large, heart-shaped leaves and purple flowers that develop into prickly seed heads, often referred to as burrs. The root itself is long, slender, and brown on the outside with a whitish flesh inside.

- **Nutritional Profile:** Burdock root is rich in nutrients, including inulin (a type of dietary fiber), antioxidants, vitamins (like vitamin C and B-complex vitamins), and minerals (such as iron, manganese, and magnesium).

- **Traditional Uses:** Burdock root has a long history of use in traditional medicine, particularly in Chinese medicine and Western herbalism. It has been used for its potential diuretic, detoxifying, and blood-purifying properties.

- **Culinary Uses:** In some cuisines, especially in Asian cooking, burdock root is used as a culinary ingredient in soups, stir-fries, and teas, prized for its earthy flavor and potential health benefits.

HEALTH BENEFITS:

1. **Detoxification Support:** Burdock root is believed to possess natural detoxifying properties. It may aid in purifying the blood by supporting the liver and kidneys, helping to eliminate toxins and metabolic waste from the body.

2. **Skin Health:** Its anti-inflammatory and antioxidant properties make burdock root beneficial for various skin conditions. It's used to alleviate skin issues like acne, eczema, psoriasis, and dry skin, promoting clearer and healthier skin.

3. **Digestive Health:** Burdock root contains inulin, a prebiotic fiber that supports the growth of beneficial gut bacteria. This fiber aids in digestion, promotes regular bowel movements, and may alleviate some digestive discomfort.

4. **Anti-inflammatory Effects:** Burdock root exhibits anti-inflammatory properties, potentially reducing inflammation throughout the body. This could be beneficial for conditions like arthritis and other inflammatory disorders.

5. **Antioxidant Activity:** It contains antioxidants that combat free radicals, reducing oxidative stress and potentially lowering the risk of chronic diseases.

6. **Immune Support:** Burdock root's compounds may have immune-strengthening effects, supporting the body's natural defenses against infections and illnesses.

7. **Diuretic Properties:** Burdock root is considered a natural diuretic, aiding in the elimination of excess fluids from the body, potentially reducing bloating and supporting kidney health.

8. **Antibacterial and Antifungal Effects:** Some studies suggest that burdock root has antibacterial and antifungal properties, which may help combat certain infections.

9. **Metabolic Health:** It's believed that burdock root may help regulate blood sugar levels, making it potentially beneficial for individuals with diabetes or those aiming to manage blood glucose levels.

Burdock root can be consumed in various forms, such as teas, tinctures, capsules, or as a culinary ingredient in soups, stir-fries, or herbal remedies. As with any herbal supplement, it's advisable to consult with a healthcare professional before incorporating burdock root into your routine, especially if you have underlying health conditions, are pregnant or breastfeeding, or are taking medications.

CALENDULA

Calendula, scientifically known as Calendula officinalis, is a bright and cheerful flowering plant that belongs to the Asteraceae or sunflower family. Commonly referred to as marigold, Calendula has been cultivated for centuries for its ornamental, culinary, and medicinal uses.

Here are key features and uses of calendula:

1. **Botanical Characteristics:** Calendula plants typically have bright orange or yellow flowers with distinctive ray and disc florets. The flowers are daisy-like in appearance and bloom throughout the growing season.

2. **Culinary Uses:** The petals of calendula flowers are edible and are sometimes used in salads, soups, and as a colorful garnish. They have a slightly peppery flavor.

3. **Medicinal Uses:** Calendula has a long history of use in traditional medicine. The flower petals are rich in flavonoids, saponins, and other compounds believed to have anti-inflammatory and healing properties.

4. **Ornamental Plant:** Beyond its practical uses, calendula is cultivated for its aesthetic appeal. Its bright and vibrant flowers make it a popular choice for gardens, borders, and floral arrangements.

Calendula is available in various forms, including dried flowers, extracts, and infused oils.

> While generally considered safe, individuals with allergies to plants in the Asteraceae family should exercise caution.

HEALTH BENEFITS

1. **Skin Healing:** Calendula is known for promoting the healing of minor wounds, cuts, and abrasions. Its application in ointments or creams may accelerate tissue repair.

2. **Anti-Inflammatory Effects:** Calendula contains compounds with anti-inflammatory properties, making it beneficial for soothing and reducing inflammation associated with skin conditions such as dermatitis.

3. **Antioxidant Properties:** The presence of antioxidants in calendula helps combat oxidative stress, protecting cells from damage caused by free radicals.

4. **Minor Burns and Sunburn Relief:** Calendula's soothing properties extend to providing relief for minor burns and sunburn. It may help calm the skin and reduce discomfort.

5. **Skin Conditions:** Calendula is used for various skin conditions, including eczema and psoriasis. Its anti-inflammatory and skin-soothing qualities make it a popular choice in natural skincare.

6. **Wound Care:** Due to its antimicrobial properties, calendula may help prevent infections in wounds, supporting the overall healing process.

7. **Menstrual Support:** In some traditional herbal practices, calendula is believed to offer support for women's health, including relief from menstrual cramps.

8. **Oral Health:** Calendula's anti-inflammatory and antimicrobial properties may be beneficial for oral health. Some toothpaste and mouthwash formulations include calendula for its potential gum health benefits.

9. **Gastrointestinal Support:** Calendula has been used traditionally to address certain gastrointestinal issues, such as indigestion and inflammation.

10. **Hair and Scalp Health:** Calendula extracts are sometimes used in hair care products for their soothing properties on the scalp and potential benefits for hair health.

It's important to note that while calendula has been used for centuries for its potential health benefits, individual responses can vary. Before using calendula for medicinal purposes, especially in concentrated forms, it's advisable to consult with a healthcare professional, particularly for individuals with allergies or sensitivities.

CAT'S CLAW

Cat's claw, also known as Uncaria tomentosa or Una de Gato, is a woody vine native to the Amazon rainforest and other areas of Central and South America. It's named for the hook-like thorns that resemble the claws of a cat. Cat's claw has been used in traditional medicine for centuries, particularly by indigenous tribes, and is known for its potential health benefits.

Key features and uses of cat's claw include:

- **Active Compounds:** Cat's claw contains various compounds, including alkaloids, flavonoids, and other phytochemicals. The two primary types of alkaloids found in cat's claw—oxindole alkaloids and quinovic acid glycosides—are believed to contribute to its medicinal properties.

- **Traditional Uses:** Indigenous communities in South America have used cat's claw for various purposes, including as a general health tonic, to treat wounds, and for its potential to support women's health.

- **Forms of Use:** Cat's claw is available in various forms, including capsules, tablets, extracts, and teas, making it convenient for consumption.

HEALTH BENEFITS:

1. **Immune Support:** Cat's claw is believed to possess immune-boosting properties, aiding in enhancing the immune system's function. It may assist in fighting infections and improving overall immune health.

2. **Anti-inflammatory Effects:** One of the most notable benefits of cat's claw is its anti-inflammatory properties. It's used to alleviate inflammation-related conditions such as arthritis, rheumatism, and other joint-related issues.

3. **Antioxidant Activity:** Cat's claw contains antioxidants that help neutralize free radicals in the body, potentially reducing oxidative stress and lowering the risk of chronic diseases.

4. **Digestive Health:** It's believed that cat's claw may support digestive health by helping to alleviate gastrointestinal issues such as gastritis, ulcers, and irritable bowel syndrome (IBS).

5. **Joint and Muscular Support:** Due to its anti-inflammatory effects, cat's claw is often used to alleviate discomfort and pain associated with various musculoskeletal conditions, including arthritis and muscle soreness.

6. **Antiviral and Antimicrobial Properties:** Some studies suggest that cat's claw exhibits antiviral and antimicrobial effects, potentially aiding in fighting certain infections and supporting the body's defense against pathogens.

7. **Wound Healing:** Cat's claw has been traditionally used topically for wound healing. Its anti-inflammatory and potential antimicrobial effects may contribute to its use in managing skin wounds.

8. **Potential Cancer Support:** Some preliminary studies have explored cat's claw's potential in cancer treatment. It's suggested that it might have properties that inhibit the growth of cancer cells, but more research is needed to validate its efficacy.

9. **Menstrual and Women's Health Support:** In traditional
    medicine, cat's claw has been used to alleviate menstrual
    discomfort and other women's health issues.

Cat's claw is available in various forms, such as capsules, tinctures, teas, and extracts. As with any herbal supplement, it's crucial to consult with a healthcare professional before using cat's claw, especially if you have existing health conditions, are pregnant or breastfeeding, or are taking medications. Additionally, the quality and dosage of herbal supplements should be carefully considered for safety and efficacy.

CAYENNE PEPPER

Cayenne pepper, also known as red pepper or Capsicum annuum, is a hot chili pepper belonging to the Capsicum genus. It's widely used as a spice in various cuisines worldwide and is known for its fiery heat and distinct flavor.

Key features and uses of cayenne pepper include:

- **Appearance:** Cayenne peppers are long, slender pods that typically range from 4 to 6 inches in length. They start as green peppers and ripen to a bright red color.

- **Heat and Flavor:** Cayenne pepper is well-known for its heat, attributed to the compound capsaicin found in its seeds and inner membranes. It has a pungent, spicy flavor that adds a fiery kick to dishes.

- **Nutritional Profile:** Cayenne pepper is low in calories and is a good source of vitamins, particularly vitamin A, vitamin C, and various antioxidants.

- **Culinary Uses:** It's used as a spice to add heat and flavor to dishes such as soups, stews, sauces, marinades, and dry rubs for meats. It's also a key ingredient in spicy cuisines like Mexican, Indian, and Thai.

HEALTH BENEFITS:

1. **Metabolism Boost and Weight Management:** Capsaicin in cayenne pepper is believed to increase metabolism and promote fat burning by generating heat in the body, potentially aiding in weight management, and supporting weight loss efforts.

2. **Appetite Suppression:** Consuming cayenne pepper may help reduce appetite by increasing feelings of fullness or satiety, which could contribute to better portion control and potentially aid in weight management.

3. **Digestive Health:** Cayenne pepper may have beneficial effects on the digestive system. It's believed to stimulate the production of digestive enzymes, promoting better digestion and nutrient absorption. However, excessive consumption can cause irritation in some individuals.

4. **Heart Health:** Some studies suggest that cayenne pepper may have cardiovascular benefits. It may help improve circulation by lowering blood pressure and supporting healthy blood flow, potentially reducing the risk of heart-related issues.

5. **Pain Relief:** Topical application of creams or ointments containing capsaicin derived from cayenne pepper may provide pain relief for conditions like arthritis, muscle aches, and nerve pain by temporarily desensitizing nerve receptors.

6. **Anti-inflammatory Effects:** Capsaicin possesses anti-inflammatory properties that may help reduce inflammation in the body, potentially benefiting conditions associated with inflammation, although more research is needed in this area.

7. **Potential Antimicrobial Properties:** Some studies indicate that capsaicin from cayenne pepper may have antimicrobial effects, potentially helping to fight certain bacterial infections.

8. **Improved Blood Sugar Control:** There's some evidence suggesting that consuming cayenne pepper may aid in managing

blood sugar levels, potentially benefiting individuals with diabetes or those aiming to control their blood glucose levels.

It's important to note that while cayenne pepper offers potential health benefits, individual responses may vary. Incorporating moderate amounts into a balanced diet may be beneficial for some individuals, but excessive consumption can cause discomfort or irritation in the digestive tract. Always consult with a healthcare professional before significantly increasing cayenne pepper intake, especially if you have existing health conditions or are taking medications.

CELTIC SEA SALT

Celtic sea salt is a type of salt that is harvested from the coastal regions of Brittany, France, near the Celtic Sea. It is often considered a more natural and less processed alternative to regular table salt. The salt is harvested through the evaporation of seawater, and it retains trace minerals and elements that are naturally found in the ocean.

Here are key characteristics and features of Celtic sea salt:

- **Harvesting Process:** Celtic sea salt is typically harvested using traditional methods that involve channeling seawater into large clay-lined basins or ponds. The sun and wind then evaporate the water, leaving behind the salt crystals.

- **Mineral Content:** One of the distinguishing features of Celtic sea salt is its mineral-rich composition. It contains a variety of trace minerals, including magnesium, calcium, potassium, and others. These minerals are believed to contribute to the salt's flavor and potential health benefits.

- **Coarse Texture:** Celtic sea salt often has a coarser texture compared to refined table salt. It may come in various grain sizes, from fine to coarse, depending on the processing method.

- **Grayish Color:** The salt's natural harvesting process, along with its mineral content, can give it a slightly grayish or off-white color. This coloration comes from the clay lining the salt ponds.

- **Distinctive Flavor:** Many people describe Celtic sea salt as having a more complex and nuanced flavor compared to regular table salt. The presence of trace minerals is believed to contribute to its unique taste.

- **Culinary Uses:** Celtic sea salt is commonly used in cooking and as a finishing salt. Its coarse texture and distinctive flavor make it a popular choice for enhancing the taste of various dishes.

- **Health Claims:** Some proponents of Celtic sea salt claim that its mineral content provides health benefits, including improved electrolyte balance, better hydration, and support for various bodily functions. However, scientific evidence supporting these claims is limited.

- **Unrefined Nature:** Unlike table salt, which often undergoes extensive processing and may have additives like anti-caking agents, Celtic sea salt is considered more natural and less refined.

HEALTH BENEFITS

1. **Trace Minerals:** Celtic sea salt contains trace minerals like magnesium, calcium, potassium, and others. These minerals play essential roles in various bodily functions, including bone health, nerve function, and electrolyte balance.

2. **Flavor Enhancement:** Celtic sea salt is praised for its unique and nuanced flavor, which can enhance the taste of dishes. Using it as a finishing salt may contribute to a more satisfying culinary experience.

3. **Reduced Sodium Intake:** Some people argue that the mineral composition of Celtic sea salt may allow individuals to achieve a desirable salty taste with less actual sodium. However, moderation in salt consumption is still crucial for overall health.

4. **Unrefined Nature:** Unlike highly processed table salt, Celtic sea salt is considered more natural and may lack additives like anti-

caking agents, making it an appealing choice for those seeking minimally processed options.

5. **Hydration Support:** Advocates suggest that the trace minerals in Celtic sea salt may contribute to better hydration by helping maintain a proper balance of electrolytes. However, scientific evidence supporting this claim is limited.

6. **Alkalizing Effect:** Some proponents claim that Celtic sea salt has an alkalizing effect on the body, potentially counteracting the acidic nature of certain foods. However, the impact of dietary salt on overall body pH is a complex topic, and more research is needed.

CHAMOMILE

Chamomile, derived from the Asteraceae family of plants, is a herb renowned for its gentle and soothing properties, primarily used in herbal medicine and as a popular ingredient in teas and skincare products. There are two main types of chamomile commonly used: German chamomile (Matricaria chamomilla or Matricaria recutita) and Roman chamomile (Chamaemelum nobile).

Key features and uses of chamomile include:

- **Appearance:** Chamomile plants have small, daisy-like flowers with white petals and a yellow center. They have a pleasant, mild fragrance.

- **Cultural History:** Chamomile has a long history of use in traditional medicine, particularly in European and Mediterranean regions. It has been utilized for its calming effects and potential health benefits.

- **Soothing Properties:** Chamomile is known for its gentle, soothing effects, often used to promote relaxation, calmness, and ease mild anxiety or stress. It's a popular choice for bedtime teas due to its calming properties.

- **Women's Health:** Chamomile tea is sometimes used to ease menstrual cramps and discomfort due to its potential muscle-relaxing properties.

- **Culinary Uses:** Chamomile flowers can be infused in hot water to make herbal tea. The tea has a mild, slightly floral taste, and it's often consumed for its calming effects.

1. **Relaxation and Stress Reduction:** Chamomile is renowned for its calming effects, which can help reduce stress and anxiety. Drinking chamomile tea or using chamomile-infused products may promote relaxation and improve overall mood.

2. **Improved Sleep Quality:** Chamomile is commonly used as a natural sleep aid. Its mild sedative effects can help improve sleep quality, making it beneficial for individuals experiencing insomnia or difficulty sleeping.

3. **Digestive Support:** Chamomile is known for its digestive benefits. It can help soothe an upset stomach, relieve gas, reduce bloating, and alleviate gastrointestinal discomfort.

4. **Anti-inflammatory Properties:** Chamomile contains compounds with anti-inflammatory effects, which can help reduce inflammation and soothe various conditions. It's often used topically to alleviate skin irritations, such as rashes, minor burns, and insect bites.

5. **Antioxidant Effects:** Chamomile is rich in antioxidants like flavonoids and terpenoids, which help combat oxidative stress and reduce the risk of chronic diseases by neutralizing free radicals in the body.

6. **Menstrual Relief:** Chamomile tea may help ease menstrual cramps and discomfort due to its potential muscle-relaxing properties.

7. **Supports Oral Health:** Rinsing with chamomile tea may contribute to improved oral health, as it possesses antimicrobial properties that could aid in reducing oral bacteria and soothing oral sores or irritations.

8. **Potential Anti-anxiety Effects:** Some research suggests that chamomile may have anxiolytic (anti-anxiety) effects, contributing to its use in managing symptoms of generalized anxiety disorder.

9. **Skin Care:** Chamomile's soothing properties make it beneficial for skincare. It's used in various skincare products to calm sensitive skin, reduce redness, and provide relief to irritated skin conditions.

Chamomile is generally considered safe for most people when consumed in moderate amounts. However, individuals allergic to plants in the Asteraceae family should use it cautiously. Pregnant or breastfeeding women and individuals taking medications should consult a healthcare professional before using chamomile supplements or products.

CHARCOAL (ACTIVATED)

Activated charcoal, also known as activated carbon, is a fine black powder made from various natural materials like coconut shells, wood, peat, or sawdust. It's processed at very high temperatures, which "activates" it by creating small pores and increasing its surface area.

Key features and uses of activated charcoal:

- **Adsorption Properties:** Activated charcoal is highly porous, with a large surface area that allows it to attract and bind to a variety of substances through a process called adsorption (not absorption). It works by binding molecules or toxins to its surface, preventing their absorption into the body.

- **Medical Uses:** In medicine, activated charcoal is used in emergency settings for certain types of poisoning or drug overdose. It's administered orally to help prevent the absorption of toxic substances in the gastrointestinal tract by binding to them and facilitating their elimination from the body through feces.

- **Water Filtration:** Activated charcoal is commonly used in water filtration systems and air purifiers due to its ability to trap impurities, chemicals, and contaminants. It helps remove odors, chlorine, volatile organic compounds (VOCs), and other pollutants from water or air.

HEALTH BENEFITS:

1. **Emergency Poisoning Treatment:** In emergency medical situations, activated charcoal is administered orally to individuals who have ingested certain toxins or drugs. It works by adsorbing

(not absorbing) toxins in the gastrointestinal tract, reducing their absorption into the bloodstream, and facilitating their elimination from the body.

2. **Relief from Digestive Discomfort:** Some people use activated charcoal supplements to potentially alleviate gas, bloating, and mild digestive discomfort. It's believed to adsorb excess gas and toxins in the digestive system, potentially reducing symptoms.

3. **Detoxification Support:** Activated charcoal is sometimes used as part of detox regimens. It's believed to help trap and eliminate toxins and impurities from the body by adsorbing them in the gastrointestinal tract.

4. **Support for Kidney Health:** In some cases, activated charcoal may be used in certain kidney-related treatments to help remove certain toxins or drugs from the bloodstream.

5. **Skincare Benefits:** Activated charcoal is an ingredient in skincare products known for its ability to draw out impurities, excess oil, and pollutants from the skin. It's used in face masks, cleansers, and soaps to promote clearer skin.

6. **Water and Air Filtration:** Activated charcoal is used in water filtration systems and air purifiers due to its adsorption properties. It helps remove impurities, chemicals, odors, and pollutants from water and air.

7. **Teeth Whitening:** Activated charcoal is occasionally used in DIY teeth whitening remedies. Its abrasive nature and adsorption properties are believed to remove surface stains from teeth, although its long-term safety and effectiveness for this purpose are debated.

While activated charcoal offers various potential benefits, its use should be approached cautiously. It can interfere with the absorption of medications and nutrients in the body and may have side effects, including constipation or vomiting. Consulting with a healthcare professional before using activated charcoal supplements or for medicinal purposes is recommended, especially if you have specific health conditions or are taking medications. Additionally, always ensure you're using food-grade or medicinal-grade activated charcoal for any oral consumption.

CILANTRO

Cilantro, also known as coriander (Coriandrum sativum), is an herb that's widely used in various cuisines around the world for its distinctive flavor and aroma. Both the leaves and seeds of the cilantro plant are utilized in cooking and have unique characteristics.

Here are key features and uses of cilantro:

- **Appearance:** Cilantro leaves, also called coriander leaves, are flat and lacy, resembling parsley, with a bright green color. The plant produces small white or pale pink flowers, and the seeds, known as coriander seeds, are round and beige in color.

- **Flavor Profile:** Cilantro leaves have a fresh, citrusy, and slightly peppery flavor. Some describe its taste as a combination of parsley and citrus. Coriander seeds have a warm, aromatic, and slightly citrusy flavor.

- **Nutritional Content:** Cilantro leaves are rich in vitamins (especially vitamin K and vitamin A), minerals, and antioxidants. They also contain essential oils that contribute to their distinct flavor.

- **Health Benefits:** Cilantro is believed to have some health benefits. It's thought to have antioxidant properties that may help protect against oxidative stress. Some studies suggest it may have potential chelating properties, aiding in the removal of heavy metals from the body.

- **Freshness:** Cilantro is best used fresh, as its flavor diminishes when cooked or dried. It's often added to dishes just before serving to retain its vibrant flavor.

❧ **Versatility:** Cilantro is a versatile herb that pairs well with a wide range of ingredients, adding a burst of freshness and depth to various dishes.

HEALTH BENEFITS:

1. **Rich in Nutrients:** Cilantro leaves are packed with vitamins and minerals, including vitamin K, vitamin A, vitamin C, folate, potassium, and manganese. These nutrients play essential roles in various bodily functions, such as immune health, bone health, and antioxidant defense.

2. **Antioxidant Properties:** Cilantro contains antioxidants like flavonoids, phenolic compounds, and carotenoids. These antioxidants help combat oxidative stress by neutralizing free radicals in the body, potentially reducing the risk of chronic diseases.

3. **Potential Heavy Metal Detoxification:** Some studies suggest that cilantro may have chelating properties, aiding in the removal of heavy metals like lead, mercury, and aluminum from the body. This property is under research and not yet fully established.

4. **Digestive Health:** Cilantro may promote digestive health due to its fiber content. It may help prevent constipation and support healthy digestion by promoting bowel regularity.

5. **Anti-inflammatory Effects:** Some components in cilantro exhibit anti-inflammatory properties that may help reduce inflammation in the body. This could potentially benefit conditions linked to inflammation.

6. **Possible Antibacterial and Antifungal Effects:** Cilantro contains compounds that have shown antibacterial and antifungal activities in some studies, suggesting potential benefits in combating certain microbial infections.

7. **Heart Health Support:** The antioxidants and other bioactive compounds in cilantro may contribute to heart health by reducing oxidative stress, which is a contributing factor to heart disease.

8. **Skin Health:** Topical applications or extracts of cilantro may have benefits for skin health. Its antioxidants and potential anti-inflammatory effects might help soothe skin irritations and promote healthier skin.

9. **Regulation of Blood Sugar Levels:** Some research suggests that cilantro may help regulate blood sugar levels, potentially benefiting individuals with diabetes or those aiming to manage blood glucose levels.

CINNAMON

Cinnamon is a highly prized spice derived from the inner bark of several tree species from the genus Cinnamomum. It's known for its sweet, warm, and aromatic flavor, making it a popular ingredient in both sweet and savory dishes as well as beverages.

Here are some key features and uses of cinnamon:

- **Varieties:** There are different types of cinnamon, with the most common being Cassia cinnamon (Cinnamomum cassia) and Ceylon cinnamon (Cinnamomum verum or Cinnamomum zeylanicum). Cassia cinnamon is more commonly found and has a stronger, slightly bittersweet taste compared to the sweeter and more delicate Ceylon cinnamon.

- **Flavor Profile:** Cinnamon has a distinct sweet and woody flavor with aromatic notes. It adds warmth and depth to dishes and is often used in both sweet recipes (like desserts, pastries, and beverages) and savory dishes (such as curries, stews, and marinades).

- **Appearance:** Cinnamon sticks are rolled or curled bark pieces, while ground cinnamon is made by grinding the bark into a powder. The color ranges from light reddish-brown to dark brown, depending on the type and quality.

- **Nutritional Content:** Cinnamon contains antioxidants, including polyphenols, which help combat oxidative stress in the body. It's also a source of manganese, iron, and calcium, albeit in small amounts.

- **Health Benefits:** Cinnamon has been associated with several potential health benefits. It may help regulate blood sugar levels by improving insulin sensitivity and reducing blood sugar spikes after meals. Some studies suggest that it may have anti-inflammatory and antimicrobial properties as well.

- **Aromatherapy and Potpourri:** Cinnamon's pleasant aroma makes it a popular choice for aromatherapy and as an ingredient in potpourri to create a warm and inviting atmosphere.

- **Traditional Medicine:** In some cultures, cinnamon has been used in traditional medicine to help alleviate digestive issues, such as indigestion and gas.

- **Culinary Uses:** Cinnamon is a versatile spice used in a wide range of dishes, including baked goods like cinnamon rolls, apple pie, oatmeal, spiced beverages (like mulled wine or chai tea), and various savory dishes in Middle Eastern, Indian, and Southeast Asian cuisines.

HEALTH BENEFITS:

1. **Antioxidant Properties:** Cinnamon is rich in antioxidants, such as polyphenols, which help protect the body from oxidative stress. These antioxidants may help reduce inflammation and combat oxidative damage caused by free radicals.

2. **Blood Sugar Regulation:** Cinnamon may have a positive impact on blood sugar levels. Studies suggest that it can improve insulin sensitivity and help lower blood sugar levels by reducing insulin resistance, potentially benefiting individuals with type 2 diabetes or those aiming to manage blood glucose levels.

3. **Anti-inflammatory Effects:** Some compounds in cinnamon exhibit anti-inflammatory properties, which may help reduce inflammation in the body. Chronic inflammation is linked to various health conditions, and cinnamon's anti-inflammatory effects could potentially offer benefits in managing related issues.

4. **Antimicrobial and Antifungal Activity:** Cinnamon contains compounds that possess antimicrobial and antifungal properties, potentially aiding in fighting certain bacterial and fungal infections.

5. **Heart Health Support:** Some research suggests that cinnamon may contribute to heart health by lowering LDL (bad) cholesterol levels and triglycerides, thereby reducing the risk factors associated with cardiovascular diseases.

6. **Neuroprotective Effects:** There is ongoing research suggesting that cinnamon might have neuroprotective effects, potentially aiding in the protection of brain health and reducing the risk of neurodegenerative diseases.

7. **Digestive Health:** Traditionally, cinnamon has been used to aid digestion. It may help alleviate digestive discomfort, such as bloating and gas, by promoting healthy digestion and soothing the gastrointestinal tract.

8. **Potential Cancer-Fighting Properties:** Some studies indicate that cinnamon's compounds may have anti-cancer effects, but more research is needed to establish its efficacy in preventing or treating cancer.

It's important to note that while cinnamon offers potential health benefits, individual responses may vary. However, excessive intake of certain types of cinnamon, particularly Cassia cinnamon, should be avoided due to higher coumarin content, which could be harmful in large doses. As with any dietary addition or supplement, consulting with a healthcare professional is advisable, especially if you have underlying health conditions or are taking medications.

COPTIS (GOLDTHREAD)

Coptis is a genus of flowering plants belonging to the Ranunculaceae family. One of the well-known species within this genus is Coptis chinensis, commonly known as Chinese goldthread or Huang Lian in Chinese. This plant has been used in traditional Chinese medicine for its medicinal properties. Here are key features of Coptis:

- **Botanical Characteristics:** Coptis plants are herbaceous perennials with small, lobed leaves and delicate, often inconspicuous flowers. The plants typically grow in cool, damp, and mountainous regions.

- **Medicinal Uses:** Coptis chinensis, in particular, has a long history of use in traditional Chinese medicine. The rhizomes (underground stems) of the plant are the primary medicinal part. They are often harvested, dried, and used for various health purposes.

- **Active Compounds:** Coptis contains several bioactive alkaloids, with berberine being one of the most prominent. Berberine is recognized for its potential antimicrobial, anti-inflammatory, and antioxidant properties.

- **Traditional Applications:** In traditional Chinese medicine, Coptis has been used to address digestive issues, including diarrhea and gastrointestinal infections. It is also employed for its potential to clear heat and dampness from the body.

1. **Digestive Health Support:** Coptis is traditionally used in traditional Chinese medicine to address digestive issues, including diarrhea and gastrointestinal infections.

2. **Antibacterial Properties:** The active compound berberine found in Coptis exhibits antibacterial effects, making it potentially useful for combating certain bacterial infections.

3. **Antiviral Properties:** Berberine has been studied for its antiviral properties, suggesting it may have potential benefits in addressing certain viral infections.

4. **Anti-Inflammatory Effects:** Coptis, particularly its constituent berberine, has demonstrated anti-inflammatory effects, which may contribute to its potential benefits in inflammatory conditions.

5. **Cardiovascular Health:** Research indicates that berberine may have cardiovascular benefits, including its potential to positively impact cholesterol levels and blood pressure.

6. **Liver Protection:** Coptis is used in traditional medicine for liver support, and berberine has been studied for its potential protective effects on the liver.

7. **Skin Health:** Due to its antimicrobial and anti-inflammatory properties, Coptis or berberine-containing preparations are sometimes used for certain skin conditions.

8. **Metabolic Support:** Berberine has been explored for its potential to support metabolic health, including its impact on weight management and insulin sensitivity.

9. **Gastrointestinal Inflammation:** Coptis may have benefits in addressing gastrointestinal inflammation, contributing to its traditional use for various digestive issues.

10. **Blood Sugar Regulation:** Berberine found in Coptis has been investigated for its ability to help regulate blood sugar levels.

It's important to note that while Coptis and its active compound berberine show promise in these areas, more research is needed to establish their efficacy and safety conclusively.

Corydalis is a genus of flowering plants belonging to the poppy family (Papaveraceae). These plants are known for their distinctive, often tubular-shaped flowers and finely divided leaves. One species within this genus, Corydalis yanhusuo, has been used in traditional Chinese medicine for its potential medicinal properties. Here are key features and aspects of Corydalis:

- **Botanical Characteristics:** Corydalis plants can vary in size and appearance, but they typically have delicate, fern-like leaves and unique spurred flowers that come in various colors, including shades of yellow, pink, and purple.

- **Medicinal Uses:** Corydalis yanhusuo, in particular, is valued in traditional Chinese medicine for its rhizomes, which are the underground stems. The rhizomes are harvested, dried, and often used in herbal formulations.

- **Active Compounds:** Corydalis contains alkaloids, with dehydrocorybulbine (DHCB) and corydine being notable constituents. These alkaloids are believed to contribute to the plant's potential medicinal effects.

- **Pain Relief:** In traditional Chinese medicine, Corydalis is used for its potential analgesic (pain-relieving) properties. It has been employed to address various types of pain, including menstrual pain and abdominal discomfort.

1. **Analgesic Properties:** Corydalis has been traditionally used for its potential to relieve pain, including menstrual pain and abdominal discomfort.

2. **Anti-Inflammatory Effects:** Compounds in Corydalis, such as alkaloids, may exhibit anti-inflammatory properties, making it of interest for conditions involving inflammation.

3. **Cardiovascular Health:** Research has explored the cardiovascular effects of Corydalis, including its potential to relax blood vessels, contributing to its traditional use for cardiovascular health.

4. **Antispasmodic Action:** Corydalis has been used as an antispasmodic agent, potentially helping to relax muscles and alleviate muscle cramps.

5. **Sedative and Anxiolytic Effects:** Some traditional uses of Corydalis involve its potential to induce relaxation and reduce anxiety.

6. **Respiratory Support:** Corydalis is sometimes used in traditional herbal practices for respiratory conditions, such as coughs and chest discomfort.

7. **Traditional Chinese Medicine (TCM):** Corydalis is a common herb in TCM formulations, tailored to individual symptoms and patterns within the framework of traditional Chinese medical diagnosis.

8. **Smooth Muscle Relaxation:** Corydalis may have the ability to relax smooth muscles, which could have implications for various bodily functions.

9. **Neuroprotective Properties:** Some studies suggest that Corydalis may have neuroprotective effects, potentially protecting nerve cells from damage.

10. **Mood Regulation:** Corydalis has been explored for its potential to regulate mood, possibly through its sedative and calming effects.

Damiana (Turnera diffusa) is a small, aromatic shrub native to Central and South America. It belongs to the Turneraceae family and has been historically used for various medicinal and aphrodisiac purposes. Here are key features and uses of damiana:

- **Botanical Characteristics:** Damiana is a perennial shrub with small, serrated leaves and aromatic flowers. It typically grows in dry, sunny climates.

- **Traditional Uses:** Damiana has a long history of traditional use among indigenous people, particularly in Central and South America. It has been utilized as an herbal remedy for conditions such as digestive issues, respiratory problems, and as an aphrodisiac.

- **Aphrodisiac Properties:** Damiana is often reputed for its potential aphrodisiac effects. It has been traditionally used to enhance libido and sexual function, with some cultures incorporating it into rituals to promote intimacy.

- **Flavoring Agent:** Damiana has a pleasant, slightly sweet flavor. It has been used as a flavoring agent in herbal teas, liqueurs, and other beverages.

1. **Urinary Tract Health:** Damiana has been used traditionally for its potential diuretic effects, supporting urinary tract health.

2. **Rich in Antioxidants:** Damiana contains compounds with antioxidant properties, contributing to its potential ability to combat oxidative stress in the body.

3. **Mild Anxiolytic Effects:** Some studies suggest that damiana may have mild anxiolytic (anxiety-reducing) effects, making it of interest for individuals dealing with mild anxiety or nervousness.

4. **Expectorant Properties:** Damiana has been traditionally used as an expectorant, potentially aiding in the relief of respiratory conditions such as coughs and bronchitis.

5. **Mood Enhancement:** Damiana is believed to have mild mood-enhancing properties, contributing to its traditional use for promoting a sense of calm and alleviating mild stress.

6. **Respiratory Health:** Damiana has been used historically for respiratory health, addressing conditions such as coughs and bronchitis.

7. **Digestive Tonic:** In traditional herbal medicine, damiana has been utilized as a digestive tonic, assisting with issues such as indigestion and mild constipation.

8. **Traditional Aphrodisiac Use:** Damiana is reputed for its traditional use as an aphrodisiac, potentially enhancing libido and sexual function.

It's essential to note that while damiana has a history of traditional use and anecdotal reports of benefits, scientific research on its efficacy is limited. Individuals considering the use of damiana or related supplements should consult with a healthcare professional, especially if they have pre-existing health conditions or are taking medications.

DANDELION

Dandelion (Taraxacum officinale) is a common flowering plant found in many parts of the world. Despite being considered a weed by some, dandelion has a long history of use in traditional medicine and culinary practices. Nearly all parts of the dandelion plant, including its roots, leaves, and flowers, have various applications and potential health benefits.

Here are some key features and uses of dandelion:

- **Appearance:** Dandelions typically have bright yellow flowers composed of multiple tiny petals that form a round flower head. The leaves are deeply toothed and can grow in a rosette shape close to the ground.

- **Culinary Uses:** Dandelion greens are edible and have a slightly bitter taste. They are used in salads, soups, stir-fries, and teas. The flowers can be used to make dandelion wine or infused into syrups and jellies. Dandelion roots are sometimes roasted and used as a coffee substitute.

- **Nutritional Content:** Dandelion greens are rich in vitamins A, C, and K, as well as several minerals, including calcium, iron, and potassium. They also contain antioxidants and fiber, contributing to their potential health benefits.

- **Medicinal Uses:** In traditional medicine, dandelion has been used for various purposes. The roots are believed to support liver health and aid digestion. Dandelion tea or extracts from the roots or leaves are used to promote urine production as a diuretic.

1. **Nutrient-Rich:** Dandelion greens are packed with vitamins and minerals, including vitamins A, C, and K, as well as calcium, iron, and potassium. They offer a significant nutritional boost to the diet.

2. **Liver Support:** Dandelion has been traditionally used to support liver health and aid in detoxification. Compounds in dandelion roots are believed to stimulate bile production, supporting digestion and liver function.

3. **Digestive Aid:** Dandelion is considered a mild laxative and diuretic. It may help alleviate constipation and promote healthy digestion by increasing urine production and facilitating the removal of waste from the body.

4. **Anti-inflammatory Effects:** Some studies suggest that dandelion may possess anti-inflammatory properties, potentially beneficial for reducing inflammation in the body associated with various conditions.

5. **Antioxidant Activity:** Dandelion contains antioxidants that combat free radicals, reducing oxidative stress and potentially lowering the risk of chronic diseases.

6. **Potential Blood Sugar Regulation:** Some research indicates that dandelion may help regulate blood sugar levels, which could be beneficial for individuals managing diabetes or aiming to stabilize blood glucose levels.

7. **Supports Immune Health:** The high vitamin C content in dandelion leaves contributes to immune health, potentially enhancing the body's defense against infections and illnesses.

8. **Bone Health:** Vitamin K found in dandelion greens is essential for bone health and plays a role in bone mineralization, potentially contributing to overall bone strength.

9. **Skin Health:** Topical applications of dandelion extracts or oils might have benefits for skin conditions due to their potential anti-inflammatory and antioxidant properties.

10. **Diuretic Effects:** Dandelion's diuretic properties may help reduce water retention, making it useful for individuals with mild edema or bloating.

Dandelion can be consumed in various forms, including raw leaves in salads, cooked greens, teas, tinctures, or supplements. Despite its potential health benefits, individuals allergic to plants in the Asteraceae family (such as ragweed or daisies) may experience allergic reactions to dandelion. As with any herbal remedy or supplement, consulting with a healthcare professional before use is advisable, especially for individuals with existing health conditions or those taking medications.

Echinacea, also known as purple coneflower, is a flowering plant native to North America and is widely recognized for its potential health benefits, particularly in herbal medicine. The plant's roots, leaves, and flowers are commonly used in supplements, teas, and extracts for various purposes.

Here are some key features and uses of echinacea:

- **Appearance:** Echinacea plants typically have large, showy flowers with prominent spiky centers that resemble cones. The flowers can be purple, pink, white, or other shades, depending on the species.

- **Medicinal Uses:** Echinacea has a long history in traditional medicine among Native American tribes. It's commonly used as a herbal remedy to support immune health and aid in the treatment of colds, flu, and other respiratory infections.

- **Potential Cold and Flu Relief:** While research results are mixed, some studies suggest that echinacea supplements might help reduce the severity and duration of colds and flu symptoms. However, more robust scientific evidence is needed to confirm its efficacy.

- **Forms of Use:** Echinacea supplements are available in various forms, including capsules, tablets, tinctures, teas, and extracts, making it convenient for consumption.

HEALTH BENEFITS:

1. **Immune Support:** Echinacea is renowned for its ability to support the immune system. It's believed to stimulate the body's natural defense mechanisms, aiding in the prevention and management of common colds, flu, and other respiratory infections. Some studies suggest that echinacea may reduce the severity and duration of cold symptoms.

2. **Antioxidant Properties:** Echinacea contains compounds, including flavonoids and polyphenols, that act as antioxidants. These antioxidants help neutralize harmful free radicals in the body, reducing oxidative stress and potentially lowering the risk of chronic diseases.

3. **Anti-inflammatory Effects:** Echinacea may possess anti-inflammatory properties, although the extent and specific mechanisms of its anti-inflammatory effects require further scientific investigation. It's believed to help reduce inflammation in the body, potentially benefiting conditions associated with inflammation.

4. **Wound Healing:** Topical applications of echinacea, such as creams or ointments, are used for their potential wound-healing properties. They might aid in skin regeneration and alleviate minor skin irritations or infections.

5. **Respiratory Health:** Echinacea is often used to support respiratory health. It's believed to ease symptoms of respiratory infections, coughs, and sore throats.

6. **Potential Antiviral and Antibacterial Effects:** Some research suggests that echinacea may possess antiviral and antibacterial properties, contributing to its use in combating certain infections.

7. **Adaptogenic Effects:** Echinacea is considered an adaptogen, a substance that helps the body adapt to stressors. It might support

the body's resilience and response to stress, potentially contributing to overall well-being.

8. **Skin Health:** Echinacea extracts might be beneficial for skin health due to their potential antimicrobial and anti-inflammatory effects. They could aid in managing certain skin conditions or promoting skin recovery.

While echinacea offers potential health benefits, individual responses can vary. It's advisable to use echinacea supplements or products cautiously and under the guidance of a healthcare professional, especially if you have existing health conditions, are pregnant or breastfeeding, or are taking medications. Additionally, more research is needed to fully understand and confirm its efficacy in various health applications.

ELDERBERRY

Elderberry refers to the dark purple berries of the elder tree (Sambucus nigra), a flowering plant native to Europe, North America, and parts of Asia. These berries have been used for centuries in traditional medicine and culinary practices due to their potential health benefits and rich nutritional profile.

Here are some key features and uses of elderberry:

- **Appearance:** Elderberries are small, dark purple berries that grow in clusters on the elder tree. They are typically harvested when ripe and can be consumed fresh, although they are often processed into juices, syrups, jams, or supplements.

- **Nutritional Content:** Elderberries are rich in vitamins, particularly vitamin C and dietary fiber. They also contain flavonoids, phenolic compounds, and antioxidants, contributing to their potential health-promoting properties.

- **Health Benefits:** Elderberries are renowned for their potential immune-boosting properties. They are commonly used as a natural remedy to support the immune system, particularly during cold and flu seasons. Some studies suggest that elderberry extracts may help reduce the severity and duration of cold and flu symptoms.

- **Culinary Uses:** Elderberries are used to make various products, including elderberry syrup, jams, jellies, and wines. They are also used in baking, cooking, and herbal teas.

HEALTH BENEFITS:

1. **Immune Support:** Elderberries are prized for their immune-boosting properties. They contain compounds that may help stimulate the immune system, potentially reducing the severity and duration of colds, flu, and other respiratory infections. Some studies suggest elderberry extracts may enhance immune response and reduce symptoms.

2. **Antioxidant Activity:** Elderberries are rich in antioxidants, including flavonoids and phenolic compounds. These antioxidants help neutralize free radicals, reducing oxidative stress and protecting cells from damage. The high antioxidant content may contribute to overall health and lower the risk of chronic diseases.

3. **Anti-inflammatory Effects:** Compounds in elderberries have demonstrated potential anti-inflammatory properties. They may help reduce inflammation in the body, potentially benefiting conditions linked to inflammation, such as arthritis and certain inflammatory disorders.

4. **Respiratory Health:** Elderberry syrup or extracts are commonly used to alleviate respiratory symptoms associated with colds, coughs, congestion, and sore throats. They are believed to have soothing effects on the respiratory tract.

5. **Heart Health:** The antioxidants in elderberries may contribute to heart health by reducing oxidative stress and inflammation. They might help support cardiovascular health by improving blood vessel function and reducing the risk of heart-related issues.

6. **Antiviral and Antibacterial Effects:** Some studies suggest that elderberry extracts may have antiviral and antibacterial properties, potentially aiding in fighting certain viruses and bacteria.

7. **Potential Skin Benefits:** Elderberry extracts or oils might have benefits for skin health due to their antioxidant and anti-

inflammatory properties. They may help soothe skin irritations and support overall skin health.

8. **Cognitive Health:** There is emerging research suggesting that the antioxidants in elderberries might have potential benefits for cognitive health by protecting against oxidative stress in the brain.

Elderberries are commonly consumed in processed forms like syrups, extracts, or supplements. While elderberries offer potential health benefits, it's advisable to use commercially prepared elderberry products and consult with a healthcare professional before use, especially if you have underlying health conditions, are pregnant or breastfeeding, or are taking medications.

EUCOMMIA

Eucommia, scientifically known as Eucommia ulmoides, is a deciduous tree native to China. It belongs to the family Eucommiaceae and is commonly referred to as "hardy rubber tree" or "Du Zhong" in traditional Chinese medicine (TCM). The tree is notable for its unique combination of medicinal and industrial uses. Here are key features and uses of Eucommia:

- **Botanical Characteristics:** Eucommia is a medium-sized tree with simple, serrated leaves and a grayish-brown bark. It is dioecious, meaning there are separate male and female trees.

- **Cultural and Traditional Significance:** Eucommia holds cultural significance in China and has been cultivated for centuries. It is considered a valuable medicinal plant in TCM.

- **Medicinal Uses:** The bark of Eucommia is the primary medicinal part. It has been traditionally used in TCM for its potential to tonify the kidneys and liver, strengthen the bones and muscles, and support overall vitality.

- **Industrial Uses:** Apart from its medicinal properties, Eucommia is cultivated for its latex, which has rubber-like qualities. However, the latex production is not as extensive as that of rubber trees, limiting its industrial use.

HEALTH BENEFITS

1. **Latex Production:** Eucommia is cultivated for its latex, which has rubber-like qualities. Although its latex production is not as extensive as that of rubber trees, it is one of the notable industrial uses of the tree.

2. **Traditional Adaptogen:** In traditional Chinese medicine, Eucommia is classified as an adaptogen, believed to help the body adapt to stress and promote overall well-being.

3. **Anti-Hypertensive Effects:** Eucommia has been studied for its potential anti-hypertensive properties, suggesting it may contribute to the regulation of blood pressure.

4. **Potential Metabolic Benefits:** Some studies suggest that Eucommia may have metabolic benefits, including its potential to regulate glucose and lipid metabolism.

5. **Bone and Joint Health:** Traditional uses of Eucommia include its application for promoting bone and joint health. It is believed to strengthen the skeletal system and alleviate conditions like arthritis.

6. **Anti-Inflammatory Effects:** Eucommia has been explored for its anti-inflammatory properties, potentially contributing to its traditional use for conditions involving inflammation.

7. **Antioxidant Activity:** Eucommia contains compounds with antioxidant properties, helping to neutralize free radicals in the body.

Individuals considering the use of Eucommia or related supplements should consult with a healthcare professional, especially if they have pre-existing health conditions or are taking medications.

FEVERFEW

Feverfew (Tanacetum parthenium) is a herbaceous plant belonging to the Asteraceae family. Native to the Balkan Peninsula, it is now widespread and cultivated in various parts of the world. Feverfew has a long history of use in traditional medicine, particularly for its potential medicinal properties. Here are key features and uses of feverfew:

- **Botanical Characteristics:** Feverfew is a perennial herb that grows up to two feet in height. It has bright green, citrus-scented, and deeply lobed leaves. The plant produces clusters of small, daisy-like flowers with white petals and yellow centers.

- **Medicinal Uses:** Feverfew has been traditionally used for various medicinal purposes, especially in folk medicine and traditional herbal practices. It gained popularity for its potential to alleviate symptoms associated with fevers and migraines.

- **Active Compounds:** The active compounds in feverfew include parthenolide and other sesquiterpene lactones. Parthenolide is believed to be responsible for the herb's anti-inflammatory and medicinal effects.

HEALTH BENEFITS

1. **Migraine Prevention:** Feverfew has been studied for its potential to prevent migraines and reduce the frequency and severity of migraine attacks.

2. **Anti-Inflammatory Properties:** Feverfew contains active compounds, such as parthenolide, known for their anti-inflammatory effects. This may make it beneficial for conditions associated with inflammation.

3. **Arthritis Support:** Due to its anti-inflammatory properties, feverfew has been explored for its potential benefits in supporting individuals with arthritis, helping to reduce inflammation and alleviate symptoms.

4. **Fever Reduction:** Historically, feverfew has been used to lower fevers, reflecting its traditional use as a remedy for fever.

5. **Digestive Aid:** Feverfew has been used to address digestive issues, including indigestion and bloating, although its primary use is more associated with its effects on headaches and inflammation.

6. **Menstrual Support:** Some women use feverfew to alleviate symptoms associated with menstruation, such as cramps and discomfort.

7. **Skin Conditions:** The anti-inflammatory properties of feverfew have led to its use in traditional medicine for certain skin conditions, including minor irritations.

It's important to note that while feverfew has been traditionally used for various purposes, its efficacy and safety should be approached with caution. Individual responses may vary, and consulting with a healthcare professional.

FO-TI

Fo-ti, also known as Polygonum multiflorum or He Shou Wu, is a perennial climbing plant belonging to the buckwheat family, Polygonaceae. Native to China, fo-ti has been used for centuries in traditional Chinese medicine (TCM) for its potential health benefits. Here are key features and uses of fo-ti:

- **Botanical Characteristics:** Fo-ti is a herbaceous vine with heart-shaped leaves and red stems. It produces clusters of small, white to pale pink flowers. The roots of the plant are the most commonly used part in traditional medicine.

- **Traditional Uses:** Fo-ti has a long history of use in TCM, where it is often known as "He Shou Wu," named after a Chinese man who reputedly restored his vitality and darkened his gray hair by using the herb.

- **Tonic and Adaptogenic Properties:** In TCM, fo-ti is considered an adaptogen and a tonic herb. It is traditionally used to tonify the liver and kidneys, nourish the blood, and promote overall vitality and longevity.

1. **Anti-Aging Properties:** Fo-ti is traditionally associated with anti-aging benefits, believed to promote longevity and maintain youthful qualities.

2. **Hair Health:** Fo-ti is used in traditional medicine to support hair health, prevent premature graying, and promote hair growth.

3. **Reproductive Health:** In traditional Chinese medicine, fo-ti is sometimes employed to support reproductive health and enhance libido. It is believed to tonify the reproductive organs.

4. **Liver and Kidney Tonification:** Fo-ti is considered a tonic herb in TCM, traditionally used to tonify the liver and kidneys, promoting overall vitality.

5. **Immune System Support:** Some traditional uses of fo-ti include its potential to support the immune system, enhancing the body's resistance to stressors.

6. **Antioxidant Properties:** Fo-ti contains compounds with antioxidant properties, which may help neutralize free radicals and protect cells from oxidative damage.

7. **Cardiovascular Health:** Traditional uses of fo-ti include its potential benefits for cardiovascular health, supporting healthy blood circulation and heart function.

8. **Digestive Health:** Fo-ti is sometimes used in traditional medicine to support digestive health, addressing issues such as constipation and promoting a healthy digestive system.

It's important to note that while fo-ti has a rich history of traditional use, scientific research on its efficacy is limited, and individual responses may vary. Consultation with a healthcare professional is advisable before using fo-ti for medicinal purposes, especially if you have pre-existing health conditions or are taking medications.

GARLIC

Garlic (Allium sativum) is a widely used and highly valued herb known for its distinctive aroma, flavor, and numerous health benefits. It's a member of the onion genus and has been utilized for culinary and medicinal purposes for thousands of years.

Here are some key features and uses of garlic:

- **Appearance:** Garlic is composed of multiple cloves clustered together in a bulb. Each clove is covered by a papery skin. The cloves can vary in size and color, typically white or off-white.

- **Flavor and Aroma:** Garlic has a pungent and savory taste with a strong, distinctive aroma. When cooked, it transforms into a milder and sweeter flavor, making it a versatile ingredient in various cuisines.

- **Culinary Uses:** Garlic is a staple ingredient in cooking worldwide. It's used to flavor savory dishes, including soups, sauces, stir-fries, marinades, roasted vegetables, and meats. It's also used raw in dressings, dips, and spreads.

- **Nutritional Content:** Garlic is low in calories but rich in nutrients. It contains vitamins C and B6, manganese, selenium, and trace amounts of other nutrients. Allicin, a sulfur compound found in garlic, is believed to be responsible for many of its health benefits.

- **Medicinal Properties:** Garlic has been used in traditional medicine for its potential medicinal properties. It's believed to have antibacterial, antifungal, and antiviral properties, potentially aiding in combating infections.

1. **Heart Health:** Garlic is linked to cardiovascular benefits. It may help lower blood pressure by promoting blood vessel dilation, potentially reducing the risk of heart disease and stroke. Additionally, garlic may help lower LDL cholesterol levels and improve overall cholesterol profile.

2. **Antioxidant Properties:** Garlic contains antioxidants, such as allicin, which help neutralize free radicals in the body. These antioxidants play a role in reducing oxidative stress and preventing cellular damage linked to chronic diseases and aging.

3. **Immune Support:** Garlic is believed to have immune-boosting properties due to its antibacterial, antiviral, and antifungal properties. It may help the body fight infections and support immune function, potentially reducing the severity and duration of colds and flu.

4. **Anti-inflammatory Effects:** Compounds in garlic have been studied for their potential anti-inflammatory properties. Garlic may help reduce inflammation in the body, benefiting conditions linked to inflammation, such as arthritis and certain inflammatory disorders.

5. **Cancer Prevention:** Some research suggests that garlic consumption might be associated with a reduced risk of certain cancers, particularly those affecting the digestive system, such as stomach and colon cancer. However, more research is needed to confirm its effectiveness.

6. **Digestive Health:** Garlic has prebiotic properties that can promote the growth of beneficial gut bacteria, contributing to digestive

health and potentially aiding in maintaining a healthy gut microbiome.

7. **Detoxification:** Garlic may support detoxification processes in the body by aiding in the elimination of toxins and heavy metals.

8. **Respiratory Health:** Garlic's antimicrobial properties might assist in alleviating respiratory infections, coughs, and sore throats. It's often used as a natural remedy for respiratory issues.

9. **Bone Health:** Some studies suggest that garlic might have a protective effect on bone health by increasing estrogen levels in females, potentially reducing the risk of osteoporosis.

10. **Skin Benefits:** Garlic's antibacterial and antifungal properties could benefit skin health, aiding in managing acne, fungal infections, and other skin conditions.

While garlic offers numerous potential health benefits, it's essential to consume it as part of a balanced diet rather than relying solely on supplements. Always consult with a healthcare professional before making significant dietary changes or starting new supplements, especially if you have existing health conditions or are taking medications.

GINGER

Ginger (Zingiber officinale) is a flowering plant whose rhizome, or underground stem, is widely used as a spice and for its medicinal properties. This aromatic herb is highly valued for its unique flavor, culinary versatility, and various health benefits.

Here are key features and uses of ginger:

- **Appearance:** Ginger rhizomes have a knobby and irregular shape with a pale yellowish or light brown skin. The flesh inside can range from ivory to yellow and is juicy with a fibrous texture.

- **Flavor and Aroma:** Ginger has a warm, spicy, and slightly sweet flavor with a peppery and citrusy aroma. It adds a distinctive and refreshing taste to dishes.

- **Culinary Uses:** Ginger is a popular spice in cuisines worldwide. It's used fresh, dried, powdered, or in the form of an extract or oil. It's a versatile ingredient in savory dishes, soups, stir-fries, marinades, baked goods, teas, and beverages like ginger ale and ginger tea.

- **Medicinal Properties:** Ginger has been used for centuries in traditional medicine for its potential health benefits. It contains bioactive compounds like gingerol and shogaol that contribute to its medicinal properties.

HEALTH BENEFITS:

1. **Digestive Health:** Ginger is well-known for its digestive properties. It aids digestion by stimulating the production of digestive enzymes and bile, which helps break down food and alleviate digestive discomfort, bloating, gas, and indigestion.

2. **Nausea Relief:** Ginger is effective in reducing nausea and vomiting, especially in cases of motion sickness, morning sickness during pregnancy, or post-operative nausea. It's commonly used as a natural remedy to alleviate these symptoms.

3. **Anti-inflammatory Effects:** Ginger contains bioactive compounds, such as gingerol and shogaol, which possess anti-inflammatory properties. These compounds may help reduce inflammation in the body, potentially benefiting conditions like osteoarthritis, rheumatoid arthritis, and muscle soreness.

4. **Pain Relief:** Some studies suggest that ginger may have analgesic properties and can help alleviate various types of pain, including menstrual pain, headaches, and muscle discomfort.

5. **Antioxidant Activity:** Ginger is rich in antioxidants that combat oxidative stress by neutralizing free radicals. These antioxidants may help protect cells from damage and reduce the risk of chronic diseases.

6. **Immune Support:** Ginger's antimicrobial properties may help strengthen the immune system, providing defense against infections and contributing to overall immune health.

7. **Cardiovascular Health:** Ginger may have cardiovascular benefits by potentially lowering cholesterol levels and blood pressure. It might also help improve blood circulation, reducing the risk of heart disease.

8. **Potential Cancer-Fighting Properties:** Some studies suggest that ginger contains compounds that could inhibit the growth of certain

cancer cells. However, further research is needed to confirm its efficacy in cancer prevention or treatment.

9. **Blood Sugar Regulation:** Preliminary research indicates that ginger might help regulate blood sugar levels and improve insulin sensitivity, which could benefit individuals with diabetes or those aiming to manage blood glucose levels.

10. **Brain Health:** Emerging research suggests that ginger's antioxidant and anti-inflammatory properties might have neuroprotective effects, potentially benefiting brain health and reducing the risk of neurodegenerative diseases.

Incorporating ginger into your diet through culinary means or as a supplement may provide these potential health benefits. However, it's important to consult with a healthcare professional, especially if you have existing health conditions or are taking medications, to determine the appropriate dosage and avoid potential interactions.

GINSENG

Ginseng refers to several species of slow-growing perennial plants belonging to the Panax genus, mainly Panax ginseng (Asian or Korean ginseng), Panax quinquefolius (American ginseng), and Panax notoginseng (Chinese ginseng). Ginseng has been used for centuries in traditional medicine, particularly in East Asia, for its potential health benefits.

Here are key features and uses of ginseng:

- **Appearance:** Ginseng plants have fleshy roots, typically with a forked shape that resembles the human body, leading to the herb's traditional use in various cultures. The roots can take several years to mature and are the main part used for medicinal purposes.

- **Varieties:** Asian ginseng (Panax ginseng) and American ginseng (Panax quinquefolius) are the most widely recognized types. They differ in their chemical composition and are used for various medicinal purposes.

- **Medicinal Properties:** Ginseng is prized for its potential health benefits and is considered an adaptogen, a substance believed to help the body adapt to stress and maintain balance. It contains active compounds called ginsenosides or panaxosides, believed to contribute to its medicinal properties.

- **Health Benefits:** Ginseng is traditionally used to boost energy, enhance cognitive function, improve mood, and support overall vitality. It's believed to enhance physical endurance and mental alertness, potentially reducing fatigue and improving focus.

1. **Boosts Energy and Reduces Fatigue:** Ginseng is believed to enhance energy levels and combat fatigue. It's commonly used to increase stamina, physical endurance, and overall vitality.

2. **Enhances Cognitive Function:** Ginseng may have cognitive benefits, including improved focus, mental clarity, and memory. It's thought to support brain health and cognitive performance, potentially benefiting attention and concentration.

3. **Stress Reduction:** Ginseng is considered an adaptogen, a substance that helps the body adapt to stressors and maintain balance. It may aid in reducing stress, supporting mental resilience, and improving overall well-being.

4. **Immune Support:** Ginseng is believed to have immune-boosting properties, assisting the body in fighting infections and strengthening the immune system against illnesses and diseases.

5. **Cardiovascular Health:** Some studies suggest that ginseng may support heart health by potentially lowering blood pressure, improving blood circulation, and reducing cholesterol levels. These effects could contribute to a lower risk of heart disease.

6. **Anti-inflammatory Effects:** Ginseng contains compounds that possess anti-inflammatory properties. It might help reduce inflammation in the body, potentially benefiting conditions linked to inflammation, such as arthritis and certain inflammatory disorders.

7. **Antioxidant Activity:** Ginseng is rich in antioxidants that help neutralize free radicals, reducing oxidative stress and protecting cells from damage. These antioxidants may contribute to overall health and lower the risk of chronic diseases.

8. **Enhances Sexual Function:** Some research suggests that ginseng might improve libido, sexual function, and erectile dysfunction in men. It's believed to have aphrodisiac properties and support reproductive health.

9. **Mood Improvement:** Ginseng may have mood-enhancing effects and could potentially alleviate symptoms of anxiety and depression, promoting mental well-being.

10. **Supports Skin Health:** Ginseng's antioxidant and anti-inflammatory properties might benefit skin health by protecting against oxidative damage and supporting skin rejuvenation.

GOLDENSEAL

Goldenseal (Hydrastis canadensis) is a perennial herb native to the eastern United States and Canada. It belongs to the Ranunculaceae family and has been historically used by Native American tribes for various medicinal purposes. Here are key features and uses of goldenseal:

- **Botanical Characteristics:** Goldenseal is a herbaceous plant with a single, hairy stem, large leaves with several lobes, and a single, greenish-white flower. The plant produces a raspberry-like fruit.

- **Rhizomes and Roots:** The medicinal part of goldenseal is its rhizomes (underground stems) and roots, which contain the plant's bioactive compounds.

- **Active Compounds:** Goldenseal contains several bioactive alkaloids, with berberine being one of the most significant. Berberine is known for its antimicrobial properties and contributes to the herb's potential medicinal effects.

- **Traditional Uses:** Goldenseal has a long history of use in traditional medicine, particularly among Native American tribes. It was traditionally used for various health purposes, including as a digestive aid and for skin conditions.

HEALTH BENEFITS

1. **Antimicrobial Properties:** Goldenseal contains berberine, which has demonstrated antimicrobial properties. It has been historically used to address infections, both topically and internally.

2. **Digestive Support:** Goldenseal has been traditionally used to support digestive health, believed to have mild laxative and appetite-stimulating effects.

3. **Immune System Support:** Some traditional uses of goldenseal include its potential to support the immune system, especially during times of illness or infection.

4. **Topical Applications:** Goldenseal is used topically for various skin conditions, wounds, and infections. It is sometimes included in herbal salves and ointments.

5. **Anti-Inflammatory Effects:** Goldenseal is believed to have anti-inflammatory properties, making it potentially beneficial for conditions involving inflammation.

6. **Respiratory Health:** Traditional uses of goldenseal include its application for respiratory health, such as addressing symptoms of colds and respiratory infections.

7. **Herbal Remedies:** Goldenseal is often included in herbal formulations, and it is sometimes used synergistically with other herbs like echinacea for immune support.

It's important to note that while goldenseal has a history of traditional use and is recognized for its antimicrobial properties, scientific research on its efficacy is limited, and individual responses may vary. Also, overharvesting has led to concerns about the conservation of wild goldenseal populations. Individuals should consult with a healthcare professional before using goldenseal for medicinal purposes, especially if they have pre-existing health conditions or are taking medications.

GOTU KOLA

Gotu kola (Centella asiatica), also known as Indian pennywort or Mandookaparni, is a perennial herb native to Asia. Widely used in traditional medicine systems, particularly in Ayurveda and traditional Chinese medicine (TCM), gotu kola has a rich history of medicinal use. Here are key features and uses of gotu kola:

- **Botanical Characteristics:** Gotu kola is a low-growing, herbaceous plant with kidney-shaped leaves and small, inconspicuous flowers. It thrives in moist, tropical environments.

- **Active Compounds:** The primary bioactive compounds in gotu kola include triterpenoid saponins, asiaticoside, asiatic acid, and madecassic acid. These compounds are believed to contribute to the herb's medicinal properties.

- **Traditional Uses:** Gotu kola has a long history of use in traditional medicine. It is considered a rejuvenating herb and has been traditionally used to support cognitive function, skin health, and overall vitality.

HEALTH BENEFITS

1. **Cognitive Support:** In traditional medicine systems like Ayurveda, gotu kola is believed to have cognitive-enhancing properties. It is considered a "brain tonic" and is used to support mental clarity and memory.

2. **Adaptogenic Qualities:** Gotu kola is often classified as an adaptogen, which means it is believed to help the body adapt to stress and promote overall well-being.

3. **Skin Health:** Gotu kola is traditionally used to promote skin health. It is believed to stimulate collagen synthesis, aiding in wound healing and potentially benefiting conditions like scars and stretch marks.

4. **Venous Insufficiency:** Some traditional uses of gotu kola involve its potential benefits for venous insufficiency, a condition where blood has difficulty returning from the legs to the heart.

5. **Anti-Inflammatory Effects:** Compounds in gotu kola, such as asiaticoside, have been studied for their anti-inflammatory properties, potentially contributing to the herb's traditional use for inflammatory conditions.

6. **Wound Healing:** Gotu kola has been traditionally used topically to aid in wound healing. It is believed to have properties that support tissue repair.

7. **Anxiolytic Effects:** Some studies suggest that gotu kola may have anxiolytic (anxiety-reducing) effects, potentially benefiting individuals dealing with mild anxiety and stress.

8. **Connective Tissue Support:** Gotu kola is believed to have a strengthening effect on connective tissues, which may be beneficial for conditions affecting ligaments, tendons, and blood vessels.

While gotu kola has a history of traditional use and some scientific studies supporting certain benefits, further research is needed to fully understand its mechanisms and efficacy. As with any herbal remedy, individuals should consult with a healthcare professional before using gotu kola for medicinal purposes, especially if they have pre-existing health conditions or are taking medications.

HOLY BASIL (TULSI)

Holy Basil, scientifically known as Ocimum sanctum or Ocimum tenuiflorum, is an aromatic herb native to the Indian subcontinent. It is also commonly referred to as Tulsi in Hindi. Holy Basil holds significant cultural, religious, and medicinal importance in various traditional systems of medicine, including Ayurveda. Here are key features and uses of Holy Basil:

- **Botanical Characteristics:** Holy Basil is a herbaceous plant with green, fragrant leaves that have a strong and distinctive aroma. The plant can grow up to about 60–90 centimeters in height and is characterized by its toothed leaves and small, purplish flowers.

- **Cultural and Religious Significance:** Holy Basil is considered a sacred plant in Hinduism and is often grown around Hindu households. It is used in religious ceremonies and is associated with various deities.

- **Medicinal Uses:** Holy Basil has a long history of medicinal use in Ayurveda, the traditional medicine system of India. It is believed to have adaptogenic, antioxidant, anti-inflammatory, and immunomodulatory properties.

- **Adaptogenic Qualities:** Holy Basil is classified as an adaptogen, which means it is believed to help the body adapt to stress and promote overall well-being.

HEALTH BENEFITS

1. **Stress Reduction:** Traditionally, Holy Basil has been used to manage stress and promote mental clarity. It is believed to have a calming effect on the nervous system.

2. **Anti-Inflammatory Effects:** Compounds in Holy Basil, such as eugenol, have demonstrated anti-inflammatory properties. This makes it potentially beneficial for conditions involving inflammation.

3. **Antioxidant Activity:** Holy Basil contains compounds with antioxidant properties, helping to neutralize free radicals in the body and protect cells from oxidative stress.

4. **Respiratory Support:** Holy Basil has been used traditionally to support respiratory health. It may be beneficial for conditions like coughs, colds, and asthma.

5. **Antimicrobial Properties:** Holy Basil is known for its antimicrobial and antibacterial properties. It has been used to address infections and promote overall immune health.

6. **Digestive Health:** Holy Basil is traditionally used to support digestive health. It may help with issues such as indigestion and bloating.

7. **Cardiovascular Health:** Some studies suggest that Holy Basil may have benefits for cardiovascular health, including its potential to regulate blood pressure and cholesterol levels.

8. **Diabetes Management:** Preliminary research indicates that Holy Basil may have a role in diabetes management by helping regulate blood sugar levels.

It's important to note that while Holy Basil has a rich history of traditional use and preliminary scientific support for certain benefits, further research is needed to fully understand its efficacy and safety. Individuals considering the use of Holy Basil for medicinal purposes should consult with a healthcare professional, especially if they have pre-existing health conditions or are taking medications.

HORNY GOAT WEED

Horny goat weed, also known as Epimedium, is an herb native to China and other parts of Asia. It has a long history of use in traditional Chinese medicine for various health purposes, particularly related to sexual health and overall well-being. The name "horny goat weed" is derived from observations that goats grazing on the plant displayed increased sexual activity.

Here are key features and uses of horny goat weed:

- **Appearance:** Horny goat weed is a flowering plant that typically grows in shaded areas and produces small, colorful flowers. It belongs to the Berberidaceae family and is characterized by its distinctive heart-shaped or oval-shaped leaves.

- **Medicinal Properties:** Horny goat weed contains active compounds such as icariin, flavonoids, and other phytochemicals believed to contribute to its potential health benefits. Icariin, in particular, is often highlighted for its role in sexual health.

- **Potential Aphrodisiac Effects:** Due to its historical use and anecdotal evidence, horny goat weed is often considered an aphrodisiac, believed to enhance sexual desire and pleasure.

- **Potential for Other Health Benefits:** While its primary use is associated with sexual health, some preliminary studies and traditional use suggest that horny goat weed might offer other health benefits, such as improving cognitive function and supporting overall vitality.

HEALTH BENEFITS:

1. **Enhanced Sexual Function:** Horny goat weed is primarily recognized for its potential in improving sexual function. It's believed to increase blood flow to the genital area, potentially aiding erectile function in men and enhancing arousal and sensitivity in women. This effect is attributed to the active compound icariin, which may function similarly to some medications used for erectile dysfunction.

2. **Libido Enhancement:** Due to its historical use as an aphrodisiac, horny goat weed is believed to boost libido and sexual desire in both men and women. It may contribute to heightened sexual interest and satisfaction.

3. **Improved Erectile Function:** Some studies suggest that horny goat weed might support erectile health by improving blood circulation and relaxing smooth muscles in the penis, potentially aiding men experiencing mild to moderate erectile difficulties.

4. **Bone Health:** Compounds in horny goat weed might have positive effects on bone density and strength. Some research indicates potential benefits for bone health, although further studies are needed to confirm these effects.

5. **Potential Antioxidant Properties:** Horny goat weed contains antioxidants that help combat oxidative stress and free radicals in the body. These antioxidants may contribute to overall health and well-being.

6. **Anti-inflammatory Effects:** Some compounds found in horny goat weed are believed to possess anti-inflammatory properties, which might be beneficial for reducing inflammation in the body and supporting joint health.

7. **Cognitive Support:** Though less studied, there's some speculation that horny goat weed may have neuroprotective effects and could

potentially support cognitive function. However, more research is needed in this area.

While horny goat weed offers potential health benefits, scientific evidence supporting its efficacy in many of these areas is limited or preliminary. It's important to consult with a healthcare professional before using horny goat weed supplements, especially if you have underlying health conditions, are taking medications, or are pregnant or breastfeeding. As with any herbal supplement, it may interact with certain medications or cause side effects in some individuals.

JIAOGULAN

Jiaogulan (Gynostemma pentaphyllum), also known as Southern Ginseng or Miracle Grass, is a herbaceous vine native to China, Japan, Korea, and certain parts of Southeast Asia. It belongs to the Cucurbitaceae family and has a long history of use in traditional Chinese medicine (TCM). Jiaogulan is known for its adaptogenic properties and potential health benefits. Here are key features and uses of jiaogulan:

- **Botanical Characteristics:** Jiaogulan is a climbing vine with small, green, and serrated leaves arranged in groups of five, resembling the leaves of ginseng, which has earned it the nickname "Southern Ginseng." The plant produces small white or greenish flowers and small, pumpkin-like fruits.

- **Adaptogenic Herb:** Jiaogulan is classified as an adaptogen, a category of herbs believed to help the body adapt to stress and promote balance.

- **Traditional Uses:** In traditional Chinese medicine, jiaogulan has been used for various health purposes, including supporting immune function, promoting longevity, and enhancing overall vitality.

HEALTH BENEFITS

1. **Antioxidant Properties:** Jiaogulan contains compounds known as gypenosides, which have antioxidant properties. Antioxidants help neutralize free radicals and protect cells from oxidative damage.

2. **Cardiovascular Health:** Some research suggests that jiaogulan may have cardiovascular benefits, including its potential to regulate blood pressure and improve lipid profiles.

3. **Immune System Support:** Traditional uses of jiaogulan include its potential to support the immune system, helping the body resist infections and illnesses.

4. **Adaptogenic Stress Response:** Jiaogulan is believed to modulate the body's response to stress, promoting a balanced and adaptive reaction to both physical and mental stressors.

5. **Respiratory Health:** Jiaogulan has been used traditionally for respiratory health, and it may have benefits for conditions like coughs and bronchitis.

6. **Anti-Inflammatory Effects:** Some studies suggest that jiaogulan may exhibit anti-inflammatory effects, potentially contributing to its traditional use for conditions involving inflammation.

7. **Digestive Health:** Jiaogulan has been used in traditional medicine to support digestive health. It may help alleviate symptoms such as indigestion and bloating.

8. **Metabolic Support:** Preliminary research indicates that jiaogulan may have metabolic benefits, including its potential to regulate blood sugar levels.

9. **Cancer Prevention:** Some studies have explored the potential anticancer properties of jiaogulan, although more research is needed to establish its efficacy in cancer prevention and treatment.

It's important to note that while jiaogulan has a history of traditional use and some scientific support for certain benefits, further research is needed to fully understand its mechanisms and efficacy. Individuals considering the use of jiaogulan for medicinal purposes should consult with a healthcare professional, especially if they have pre-existing health conditions or are taking medications.

KAVA

Kava (Piper methysticum) is a plant native to the South Pacific islands, where it has been used for centuries in traditional ceremonies and social gatherings. The root of the kava plant is used to prepare a beverage with sedative and relaxing properties. Here are key features and uses of kava:

- **Botanical Characteristics:** Kava is a member of the pepper family (Piperaceae) and is characterized by its large leaves and the thick, gnarled roots from which the kava beverage is made. The plant is primarily grown in the South Pacific region, including Fiji, Vanuatu, Tonga, and Samoa.

- **Traditional Use:** Kava has a long history of use in traditional Pacific Island cultures, particularly in social and ceremonial contexts. It is often consumed during rituals, ceremonies, and social gatherings.

- **Kava Beverage:** The traditional kava preparation involves grinding or pounding the root into a powder, which is then mixed with water to create a beverage. The active compounds in kava, known as kavalactones, are extracted during this process.

1. **Sedative and Relaxing Effects:** Kava is well-known for its sedative and relaxing properties. It is often consumed to promote a sense of calmness, relaxation, and sociability. These effects are attributed to the action of kavalactones on the central nervous system.

2. **Anxiolytic Properties:** Some people use kava as a natural remedy for anxiety and stress. Kavalactones are believed to interact with neurotransmitter receptors, producing anxiolytic (anxiety-reducing) effects.

3. **Muscle Relaxation:** Kava is known for its muscle relaxant properties. It is traditionally used to alleviate muscle tension and promote a state of physical relaxation.

4. **Mild Analgesic Effects:** In some traditional contexts, kava is used for its mild analgesic properties, helping to alleviate discomfort and pain.

5. **Varieties of Kava:** There are different varieties or cultivars of kava, each with its unique balance of kavalactones, leading to variations in taste, potency, and effects.

6. **Safety Considerations:** While kava has a long history of traditional use, there have been concerns about the potential for liver toxicity associated with certain types of kava extracts. Due to these concerns, some countries have implemented restrictions on the sale and importation of kava products. It's crucial to source kava from reputable suppliers and use it responsibly.

Individual responses to kava can vary, and excessive consumption or use of poor-quality kava may have adverse effects. It's recommended to consult with healthcare professionals before using kava, especially for individuals with liver conditions or those taking medications that may interact with kava.

LEMON BALM

Lemon balm (Melissa officinalis) is a fragrant herb belonging to the mint family (Lamiaceae). Native to Europe and Asia, it is now cultivated in various regions around the world. Lemon balm is well-known for its citrusy aroma and is valued for both culinary and medicinal purposes. Here are key features and uses of lemon balm:

- **Botanical Characteristics:** Lemon balm is a herbaceous perennial with square stems, opposite leaves, and clusters of small white or pale yellow flowers. The leaves are deeply veined and emit a lemony scent when crushed.

- **Citrus Aroma:** The leaves of lemon balm contain essential oils, including citronellal and citral, which give the plant its distinct lemon fragrance. The aroma is released when the leaves are touched or bruised.

- **Culinary Uses:** Lemon balm is used as a culinary herb to flavor a variety of dishes. It can be used fresh or dried in salads, soups, teas, and desserts. The leaves impart a mild lemon flavor to recipes.

- **Herbal Teas:** Lemon balm is commonly used to make herbal teas. The tea is known for its calming and soothing properties and is often consumed to promote relaxation and alleviate stress.

- **Medicinal Uses:** Lemon balm has been used in traditional medicine for its potential medicinal properties. It is believed to have mild sedative effects and is used to address issues like anxiety, insomnia, and digestive discomfort.

- **Culinary Garnish:** In addition to flavoring dishes, lemon balm is sometimes used as a garnish in culinary creations, adding a touch of freshness and aroma.

- **Companion Plant:** Lemon balm is considered a companion plant in gardening. It is believed to attract beneficial insects and deter certain pests.

HEALTH BENEFITS

1. **Nervine Tonic:** Lemon balm is considered a nervine tonic, meaning it has a calming and toning effect on the nervous system. It is often used to support mental well-being and ease nervous tension.

2. **Antioxidant Properties:** Lemon balm contains antioxidants, including rosmarinic acid, which may help protect cells from oxidative stress and contribute to its overall health benefits.

3. **Topical Applications:** Some use lemon balm topically in creams or salves for its potential benefits on the skin. It is believed to have soothing effects and may be applied to minor skin irritations.

4. **Cold Sores:** Lemon balm has been explored for its potential to reduce the frequency and duration of cold sores caused by the herpes simplex virus. Creams containing lemon balm extract are sometimes used for this purpose.

5. **Anti-Inflammatory Effects:** Lemon balm has been studied for its anti-inflammatory properties, which may contribute to its traditional use for conditions involving inflammation.

Lemon balm is generally well-tolerated, and its mild flavor and aromatic qualities make it a popular choice in both culinary and herbal applications. However, individuals with allergies or sensitivities should exercise caution. Before using lemon balm for medicinal purposes or in significant quantities, it's advisable to consult with healthcare professionals.

LICORICE ROOT

Licorice root, derived from the Glycyrrhiza glabra plant, has a long history of use in traditional medicine and culinary practices. It's prized for its distinct sweet flavor and various potential health benefits. Licorice root contains active compounds, such as glycyrrhizin, flavonoids, and plant sterols, which contribute to its medicinal properties.

Here are key features and uses of licorice root:

- **Appearance:** Licorice root is a woody perennial herb with a thick, woody, and fibrous root that is long and brown on the outside, with a yellowish interior. It's often used in dried or powdered form.

- **Flavor Profile:** Licorice root has a naturally sweet and slightly woody taste, often used as a flavoring agent in candies, teas, and herbal preparations.

- **Medicinal Properties:** Licorice root is recognized for its potential medicinal properties, including being anti-inflammatory, antiviral, antimicrobial, and antioxidant.

HEALTH BENEFITS:

1. **Respiratory Health:** Licorice root is used as a natural remedy for respiratory issues such as coughs, sore throats, and bronchitis. Its demulcent properties help soothe the mucous membranes in the respiratory tract, providing relief from irritation and promoting expectoration.

2. **Anti-inflammatory Effects:** Compounds found in licorice root exhibit anti-inflammatory properties, potentially benefiting conditions linked to inflammation, including arthritis, gastritis, and other inflammatory disorders.

3. **Adrenal Support:** Licorice root might support adrenal health by affecting cortisol levels in the body. It's believed to aid in stress management by supporting the adrenal glands, although prolonged or excessive use may have side effects on hormone levels.

4. **Skin Health:** Topical applications of licorice root extract or gel are used for their potential skin-soothing and anti-inflammatory effects. They may help manage skin conditions like eczema, psoriasis, and other inflammatory skin conditions.

5. **Hormonal Balance:** Licorice root may have mild estrogenic effects and is sometimes used to alleviate symptoms associated with hormonal imbalances, such as PMS (premenstrual syndrome) and menopause.

6. **Antiviral and Antimicrobial Properties:** Licorice root contains compounds with potential antiviral and antimicrobial effects, which might help combat certain viruses and bacteria. It's used in some traditional remedies for its purported immune-boosting properties.

7. **Potential for Gastric Ulcer Support:** Some studies suggest that licorice root might have protective effects on the stomach lining and could be beneficial in managing gastric ulcers, although more research is needed.

8. **Supports Liver Health:** Licorice root might have hepatoprotective properties, offering support to the liver and aiding in its detoxification processes.

9. **Weight Management:** Some studies suggest that licorice root might play a role in weight management by potentially reducing body fat, although more research is required to confirm this effect.

10. **Digestive Health:** Licorice root is known for its soothing effects on the digestive system. It may help alleviate symptoms of indigestion, heartburn, and acid reflux by coating the stomach lining and reducing inflammation. It's often used to support overall digestive health.

Despite its potential health benefits, licorice root should be used cautiously and in moderation due to the risk of side effects, especially in individuals with certain health conditions or those taking medications. It's advisable to consult with a healthcare professional before using licorice root supplements regularly.

LOMATIUM

Lomatium is a genus of flowering plants within the Apiaceae family, commonly known as the carrot or parsley family. These plants are primarily native to North America, and some species within the genus have been historically used by Native American tribes for various medicinal purposes. Here are key features and uses of Lomatium:

- **Botanical Characteristics:** Lomatium plants vary in appearance depending on the species. They generally have compound leaves, often finely divided, and produce clusters of small, umbrella-like flowers. The plants can be herbaceous perennials or shrubs.

- **Ethnobotanical History:** Several species of Lomatium have a long history of use among Native American tribes, particularly in the Western United States. Different tribes used various species for their potential medicinal properties.

- **Traditional Medicinal Uses:** Lomatium species were traditionally used for a range of ailments by indigenous peoples. The roots, in particular, were utilized in traditional medicine for their potential benefits.

HEALTH BENEFITS

1. **Respiratory Support:** Lomatium species were often used by Native American tribes to support respiratory health. Infusions or decoctions of the root were used to address respiratory conditions, including coughs and colds.

2. **Antiviral Properties:** Some Lomatium species, notably Lomatium dissectum, have been investigated for their potential antiviral

properties. Extracts from the roots have shown activity against certain viruses, although more research is needed.

3. **Immune System Support:** Traditional uses of Lomatium include its potential to support the immune system. The plant was believed to have immune-enhancing properties.

4. **Antibacterial Effects:** Certain Lomatium species have been studied for their antibacterial effects, indicating a potential role in combating bacterial infections.

5. **Anti-Inflammatory Properties:** Some research suggests that Lomatium may have anti-inflammatory properties, which could contribute to its traditional use for inflammatory conditions.

6. **Root Harvesting:** The roots of Lomatium plants are the primary part used in traditional medicine. Harvesting the roots required careful consideration to ensure sustainability and conservation of wild populations.

7. **Contemporary Herbal Use:** In modern herbalism, Lomatium extract or tincture is sometimes used to support respiratory health and immune function.

It's important to note that while Lomatium has a history of traditional use, and there is some scientific interest in its potential medicinal properties, caution is warranted. Wildcrafting and use of Lomatium should be approached with respect for conservation efforts, as overharvesting can impact wild populations. Additionally, individuals considering the use of Lomatium for medicinal purposes should do so under the guidance of a knowledgeable healthcare professional, as improper use or dosage may pose risks.

LOTUS FLOWER

The lotus flower, scientifically known as Nelumbo nucifera, is a beautiful aquatic plant that holds cultural and symbolic significance in various traditions around the world. Here are key features and characteristics of the lotus flower:

1. **Aquatic Plant:**

    - The lotus is an aquatic perennial plant that grows in various water environments, including ponds, lakes, and slow-flowing rivers.

2. **Botanical Characteristics:**

    - **Leaves:** The lotus has large, round, or oval-shaped leaves that float on the water's surface. The leaves are often held above the water, and water droplets bead on their surface due to their hydrophobic nature.

    - **Flowers:** The lotus flower is known for its exquisite beauty. It has a distinct structure with numerous petals arranged in layers, creating a symmetrical and elegant appearance.

    - **Colors:** Lotus flowers come in various colors, including white, pink, red, and blue. White and pink lotus flowers are particularly common and hold specific cultural meanings.

    - **Seed Pod:** After the lotus flower blooms, it gives rise to a unique seed pod that resembles a circular cluster of pods. These pods contain the lotus seeds.

3. **Symbolic Significance:**

- **Cultural and Religious Symbolism:** The lotus holds profound symbolism in various cultures and religions, including Hinduism, Buddhism, Jainism, and ancient Egyptian beliefs. It is often associated with purity, enlightenment, rebirth, and spiritual growth.

- **Growth from Mud:** The lotus is revered for its ability to emerge from murky, muddy waters and bloom into a pure and untarnished flower. This growth process is seen as a metaphor for spiritual awakening and enlightenment.

4. **Culinary Uses:**

- **Edible Seeds:** Lotus seeds are used in Asian cuisine and traditional medicine. They are often consumed as snacks, added to soups, or used in desserts.

5. **Aesthetic and Ornamental Uses:**

- **Gardens and Landscapes:** Lotus flowers are cultivated for their aesthetic appeal and are often grown in water gardens, ponds, and landscapes for their beauty and symbolic significance.

6. **Artistic Representation:**

- **Art and Literature:** The lotus has inspired countless works of art, literature, and poetry. Its beauty and cultural significance make it a popular subject in various creative expressions.

7. **National Flower:**

- **Symbol of Countries:** The lotus is the national flower of several countries, including India and Vietnam, where it symbolizes purity, beauty, and the strength to rise above challenges.

8. **Adaptation and Resilience:**

   - **Adaptation to Environment:** The lotus exhibits adaptations that allow it to thrive in various water conditions, from still ponds to slow-moving rivers.

The lotus flower, with its captivating beauty and rich symbolism, continues to be a source of inspiration and reverence in many cultures, religions, and artistic expressions around the world.

HEALTH BENEFITS

1. **Antioxidant Properties:** Lotus flowers and seeds contain antioxidants, which may help neutralize free radicals and protect cells from oxidative stress.

2. **Anti-Inflammatory Effects:** Compounds found in lotus plants may have anti-inflammatory properties, potentially contributing to the reduction of inflammation in the body.

3. **Digestive Aid:** In traditional medicine, lotus seeds and rhizomes have been used for their potential digestive benefits. They may have properties that aid in digestion and promote gastrointestinal health.

4. **Stress Relief and Relaxation:** Some traditional practices suggest that lotus flowers or extracts may have calming effects, contributing to stress relief and relaxation.

5. **Traditional Medicine Uses:** Various parts of the lotus plant, including the seeds and rhizomes, are used in traditional medicine systems in Asia for their potential therapeutic effects. These uses may include promoting overall well-being.

6. **Heart Health:** Some compounds in lotus plants have been studied for their potential cardiovascular benefits. This includes the potential to regulate blood pressure and improve heart health.

7. **Potential for Mental Health:** Lotus flower extracts have been explored for their potential effects on mental health, including mood enhancement and stress reduction. However, more research is needed in this area.

8. **Anti-Bacterial Properties:** Compounds in lotus plants may have antibacterial properties, which could contribute to their traditional use for certain infections or skin conditions.

9. **Anti-Aging Potential:** Antioxidants in lotus plants may play a role in protecting the skin from premature aging by preventing damage caused by free radicals.

10. **Wound Healing:** Lotus extracts have been investigated for their potential wound healing properties. Compounds found in the plant may aid in tissue repair.

It's crucial to approach the use of lotus plant components for health purposes with caution. Consultation with healthcare professionals is advisable before incorporating lotus supplements or extracts into one's diet, especially if there are existing health conditions or if the individual is taking medications. Additionally, relying on traditional uses of the lotus plant should be done with proper understanding and awareness of potential effects.

MAHONIA

Mahonia is a genus of flowering plants in the barberry family (Berberidaceae). These evergreen shrubs are known for their distinctive pinnately compound leaves, holly-like appearance, and clusters of small, fragrant flowers. Some species in the Mahonia genus are commonly cultivated as ornamental plants. Here are key features and uses of Mahonia:

- **Botanical Characteristics:** Mahonia plants are characterized by their spiny, holly-like leaves and upright, often architectural growth habit. The leaves are typically pinnately compound with several leaflets arranged along a central stem.

- **Flowers:** Mahonia plants produce clusters of small, bright yellow flowers. The flowers are often fragrant and can be borne in upright or hanging racemes.

- **Fruit:** After flowering, Mahonia plants develop grape-like clusters of berries. The berries are typically blue or black and are a key ornamental feature.

- **Evergreen Foliage:** One of the distinctive features of Mahonia is its evergreen foliage, which provides year-round interest in the landscape.

- **Ornamental Use:** Mahonia species are commonly grown as ornamental shrubs in gardens and landscapes. They are valued for their attractive foliage, flowers, and berries.

- **Landscaping:** Mahonia shrubs are often used in landscaping to create hedges, borders, or as standalone specimens. They add structure and visual interest to garden designs.

- **Drought Tolerance:** Mahonia species are generally hardy and adaptable, with some varieties exhibiting tolerance to drought conditions once established.

- **Medicinal Uses:** Some Mahonia species, particularly Mahonia aquifolium (Oregon grape), have been used in traditional herbal medicine. The roots of Oregon grape have been historically used by Native American tribes for various medicinal purposes.

- **Berberine Content:** Mahonia aquifolium is known for containing berberine, a compound with potential antimicrobial and anti-inflammatory properties. Berberine has been studied for its potential health benefits.

- **Wildlife Attraction:** The berries of Mahonia plants are attractive to birds, providing a food source in the garden. This can contribute to supporting local wildlife.

- **Cultural Significance:** In addition to their horticultural uses, Mahonia species may hold cultural significance in certain regions. For example, Mahonia aquifolium is the state flower of Oregon.

- **Tolerant of Shade:** Mahonia plants are often tolerant of shade, making them suitable for planting in areas with partial to full shade.

Common species within the Mahonia genus include Mahonia aquifolium (Oregon grape), Mahonia japonica (Japanese mahonia), and Mahonia bealei (Leatherleaf mahonia).

1. **Antimicrobial Properties:** Berberine, a compound found in Mahonia, has demonstrated antimicrobial properties. It may have activity against various bacteria, fungi, and parasites.

2. **Anti-Inflammatory Effects:** Berberine has been studied for its anti-inflammatory effects, potentially contributing to the alleviation of inflammatory conditions.

3. **Skin Conditions:** Mahonia aquifolium has been used traditionally for skin conditions such as psoriasis. Some studies suggest that topical applications of Mahonia aquifolium may help manage symptoms of certain skin disorders.

4. **Immune System Support:** Compounds in Mahonia may have immunomodulatory effects, supporting the immune system's function.

5. **Gastrointestinal Health:** Berberine has been investigated for its potential benefits in gastrointestinal health. It may help with issues such as diarrhea, bacterial infections, and inflammatory bowel conditions.

6. **Cardiovascular Health:** Some research suggests that berberine, found in Mahonia, may have cardiovascular benefits. It may help regulate cholesterol levels and support overall heart health.

7. **Blood Sugar Regulation:** Berberine has been studied for its potential to regulate blood sugar levels, making it of interest in the context of diabetes management.

8. **Antioxidant Properties:** Mahonia contains antioxidants that may help neutralize free radicals and protect cells from oxidative stress.

9. **Liver Health:** Berberine has been investigated for its potential benefits in liver health, including its role in supporting liver function and protecting against liver damage.

10. **Anti-Cancer Properties:** Some studies have explored the potential anti-cancer properties of berberine, although more research is needed to understand its efficacy in cancer prevention and treatment.

11. **Oral Health:** Berberine has been studied for its potential antibacterial effects in the oral cavity, suggesting a role in promoting oral health.

12. **Wound Healing:** Traditional uses of Mahonia include its application for wound healing. Compounds in Mahonia may have properties that support the skin's natural healing processes.

It's important to approach the use of Mahonia for medicinal purposes with caution. Berberine, while exhibiting potential health benefits, may also interact with certain medications, and excessive consumption may have side effects. Individuals with pre-existing health conditions or those taking medications should consult with healthcare professionals before using Mahonia for medicinal purposes.

MARJORAM

Marjoram (Origanum majorana) is an aromatic herb belonging to the mint family, closely related to oregano, with a delicate and sweet flavor profile. It's native to the Mediterranean region and has been utilized for culinary, medicinal, and aromatic purposes for centuries.

Here are some key features and uses of marjoram:

- **Appearance:** Marjoram is a small, bushy herb with oval-shaped, soft, gray-green leaves that grow in pairs opposite each other along the stems. It produces small clusters of tiny white or pale pink flowers when in bloom.

- **Flavor and Aroma:** Marjoram has a mild, sweet, and slightly floral flavor with hints of pine and citrus. Its aroma is fragrant and reminiscent of a blend of sweet basil and thyme, making it a versatile herb in culinary applications.

- **Culinary Uses:** Marjoram is a popular herb in Mediterranean and Middle Eastern cuisines. It's used fresh or dried to flavor various dishes, including soups, stews, sauces, roasted vegetables, meats, salads, and marinades. It complements poultry, lamb, fish, and tomato-based dishes exceptionally well.

- **Aromatic Uses:** The aromatic nature of marjoram makes it a popular ingredient in potpourris, herbal sachets, and aromatherapy. Its pleasant scent is often used for its calming and relaxing effects.

- **Topical Use:** Marjoram oil, extracted from the leaves, is sometimes used in topical applications for its potential soothing effects on muscles and joints. It might be added to massage oils or balms.

1. **Digestive Support:** Marjoram has been traditionally used to aid digestion by stimulating the digestive system. It may help relieve symptoms of indigestion, bloating, and gas, promoting overall digestive health.

2. **Respiratory Health:** Marjoram is believed to have mild expectorant properties, making it beneficial for managing minor respiratory issues like coughs, congestion, and bronchial discomfort. It's often used to ease respiratory symptoms.

3. **Anti-inflammatory Effects:** Compounds in marjoram possess anti-inflammatory properties that may help reduce inflammation in the body. This effect could potentially benefit conditions associated with inflammation, such as arthritis or muscle soreness.

4. **Antioxidant Activity:** Marjoram contains antioxidants, such as flavonoids and phenolic compounds, which help neutralize free radicals and reduce oxidative stress. These antioxidants contribute to overall health and may lower the risk of chronic diseases.

5. **Antimicrobial Properties:** Some studies suggest that marjoram exhibits antimicrobial activity against certain bacteria and fungi. It might have a role in inhibiting the growth of pathogens, contributing to immune health.

6. **Stress Relief:** Marjoram's pleasant aroma has been associated with relaxation and stress reduction. It's sometimes used in aromatherapy to promote calmness and alleviate tension.

7. **Potential Pain Relief:** Marjoram oil, when used topically, might have soothing effects on muscles and joints. It's believed to possess

analgesic properties that could aid in relieving minor aches and pains.

8. **Cognitive Health:** Some research indicates that the compounds in marjoram might have neuroprotective effects, potentially benefiting cognitive function and supporting brain health. However, more studies are needed in this area.

9. **Menstrual Support:** Marjoram is sometimes used traditionally to alleviate menstrual discomfort and cramps. It's believed to have properties that might help ease menstrual symptoms.

10. **Skin Health:** Marjoram's antioxidants and potential antimicrobial effects might have benefits for skin health, although further research is necessary to explore its specific applications in skincare.

While marjoram offers potential health benefits, it's primarily used as a culinary herb. As with any herbal remedy, consult with a healthcare professional before using marjoram for medicinal purposes, especially if you have existing health conditions, are pregnant, or are taking medications.

MILK THISTLE

Milk thistle (Silybum marianum) is a flowering herb native to the Mediterranean region and is well-known for its traditional use in herbal medicine. Its distinctive appearance, marked by spiny leaves and purple flower heads, makes it easily recognizable. The key component of milk thistle believed to impart its medicinal properties is a group of compounds collectively known as silymarin.

Here are the key features and uses of milk thistle:

1. **Appearance:** Milk thistle has large, prickly leaves with white marbling and distinctive purple flower heads that produce spiky structures of seeds. The seeds contain the active components responsible for its medicinal properties.

2. **Medicinal Properties:** The active compound, silymarin, is a flavonoid complex known for its potential hepatoprotective (liver-protecting) effects. It's believed to have antioxidant, anti-inflammatory, and liver-regenerating properties.

HEALTH BENEFITS:

1. **Liver Support:** Milk thistle is widely known for its hepatoprotective effects. Silymarin, its primary active compound, is believed to support liver health by protecting liver cells from damage caused by toxins, alcohol, pollutants, and certain medications. It may aid in liver regeneration and support overall liver function.

2. **Detoxification Aid:** Silymarin in milk thistle is thought to enhance the liver's detoxification processes by promoting the production of glutathione, a powerful antioxidant that aids in the elimination of toxins and free radicals from the body.

3. **Antioxidant Properties:** Milk thistle contains antioxidants that help neutralize free radicals, reducing oxidative stress and protecting cells from damage. These antioxidants contribute to overall health and may support various bodily functions.

4. **Digestive Health:** Some people use milk thistle to promote digestive health. Its anti-inflammatory properties might aid in soothing minor digestive issues and supporting a healthy digestive system.

5. **Cholesterol Management:** Preliminary studies suggest that milk thistle may help lower LDL ("bad") cholesterol levels. It might support cardiovascular health by potentially reducing cholesterol and triglyceride levels, although more research is needed to confirm this effect.

6. **Skin Health:** Topical applications or supplements containing milk thistle extracts are sometimes used for skin conditions like acne, eczema, and psoriasis due to its potential anti-inflammatory and antioxidant properties.

7. **Type 2 Diabetes Support:** Some research indicates that milk thistle might have a role in managing blood sugar levels in individuals with type 2 diabetes by potentially improving insulin resistance, although further studies are required to validate this effect.

8. **Potential Anti-Cancer Effects:** Studies have explored milk thistle's potential to inhibit the growth of certain cancer cells, suggesting a role in cancer prevention or treatment. However, more research is necessary to confirm its efficacy.

9. **Gallbladder Health:** Milk thistle might aid in supporting gallbladder health by promoting the flow of bile and aiding in the breakdown of fats, potentially benefiting individuals with gallbladder issues.

While milk thistle offers potential health benefits, it's essential to consult with a healthcare professional before using milk thistle supplements, especially if you have existing health conditions, are pregnant or breastfeeding, or are taking medications, as it may interact with certain drugs or have side effects in some individuals.

MINT

Mint refers to a group of aromatic herbs belonging to the Mentha genus within the Lamiaceae family, known for their refreshing aroma and various culinary, medicinal, and aromatic uses. Several mint species exist, with some of the most common varieties including spearmint (Mentha spicata) and peppermint (Mentha × piperita).

Here are the key features and uses of mint:

- **Appearance:** Mint plants typically have square-shaped stems, paired opposite leaves, and small, delicate flowers in shades of white, pink, or purple. The leaves are often smooth, serrated, and emit a strong, pleasant aroma when crushed.

- **Flavor and Aroma:** Mint has a refreshing, cool, and slightly sweet flavor with a characteristic menthol aroma. The flavor can vary among different mint varieties, with peppermint having a more intense and menthol-forward taste compared to spearmint.

- **Culinary Uses:** Mint is a versatile herb used in various culinary preparations worldwide. It adds flavor to dishes such as salads, beverages (like mint tea and mojitos), desserts, sauces, savory dishes, and as a garnish. It pairs well with fruits, chocolate, lamb, peas, and other herbs.

- **Medicinal Properties:** Mint has been used in traditional medicine for its potential health benefits. It's known for its digestive properties, helping alleviate symptoms of indigestion, gas, and bloating. Mint teas or infusions are commonly used for these purposes.

- **Aromatic Uses:** The fresh aroma of mint makes it a popular choice in aromatherapy and personal care products like soaps, lotions, and essential oils. It's believed to have uplifting and soothing effects, promoting relaxation and mental clarity.

- **Breath Freshener:** The menthol in mint makes it a popular choice for freshening breath. Chewing mint leaves or consuming mint-flavored products can help mask bad breath and leave a cooling sensation in the mouth.

- **Potential Health Benefits:** Mint is rich in antioxidants and has potential antimicrobial properties that might support overall health. It may also have soothing effects on headaches or nasal congestion due to its menthol content.

- **Gardening and Pest Control:** Mint plants are often cultivated in gardens for their easy growth and ability to repel certain pests due to their strong scent.

HEALTH BENEFITS:

1. **Digestive Health:** Mint is well-known for its digestive properties. It may help alleviate symptoms of indigestion, gas, bloating, and stomach discomfort. Mint teas or infusions are commonly used to aid digestion by promoting the flow of bile.

2. **Relief from Nausea:** The aroma and compounds in mint are believed to have a calming effect on the stomach, potentially relieving nausea and motion sickness. Chewing on fresh mint leaves or sipping mint tea might help alleviate these symptoms.

3. **Oral Health:** Mint's antibacterial properties can help freshen breath and may assist in reducing oral bacteria that contribute to

bad breath and oral infections. Some mouthwashes and toothpaste contain mint for its refreshing and antiseptic effects.

4. **Respiratory Support:** Menthol, a compound found in mint, has a soothing effect on the respiratory tract. Inhaling the steam from mint tea or using menthol-based products might help alleviate congestion and ease symptoms of colds or sinus issues.

5. **Antioxidant Properties:** Mint contains antioxidants that help neutralize free radicals in the body, reducing oxidative stress and potentially lowering the risk of chronic diseases.

6. **Headache Relief:** The cooling sensation from applying diluted mint oil or a mint-based balm on the forehead might help alleviate tension headaches and migraines due to its soothing properties.

7. **Skin Care:** Mint's anti-inflammatory and antibacterial properties might be beneficial for skin health. Topical applications of diluted mint oil may help soothe skin irritation and itching caused by insect bites or skin conditions like eczema.

8. **Mental Clarity and Relaxation:** In aromatherapy, mint's aroma is believed to enhance mental clarity, improve focus, and promote relaxation. The scent of mint might have a calming effect on the mind.

9. **Weight Management:** Some studies suggest that the aroma of mint might help reduce cravings and appetite, potentially supporting weight management efforts.

10. **Potential Anti-Cancer Properties:** Some research indicates that certain compounds in mint may have protective effects against cancer, although more studies are needed to confirm these findings.

Mint can be consumed in various forms, including fresh leaves, teas, essential oils, and incorporated into foods or beverages. It's generally considered safe for most people when consumed in moderate amounts as part of a balanced diet. However, excessive intake or concentrated forms like essential oils should be used cautiously. Individuals with specific health conditions should consult a healthcare professional before using mint for medicinal purposes.

NETTLE ROOT

Nettle root, derived from the common stinging nettle plant (Urtica dioica), has been historically used for various medicinal purposes. The root of the nettle plant is the primary part used for its potential health benefits. Here are key features and uses of nettle root:

- **Botanical Characteristics:** The stinging nettle is a perennial herbaceous plant with serrated leaves and tiny, hair-like structures on the leaves and stems that can cause a stinging sensation upon contact with the skin.

- **Root Harvesting:** The roots of the stinging nettle plant are harvested for medicinal use. They are typically collected in the fall when the plant's energy is concentrated in the roots.

- **Phytochemical Composition:** Nettle root contains various bioactive compounds, including sterols, lignans, and polysaccharides. One of the key components is beta-sitosterol, which has been studied for its potential health benefits.

HEALTH BENEFITS

1. **Anti-Inflammatory Properties:** Nettle root has been traditionally used for its anti-inflammatory properties. It is believed to help reduce inflammation, making it potentially beneficial for conditions such as arthritis.

2. **Prostate Health:** Nettle root is often used in herbal remedies targeting prostate health. Some studies suggest that nettle root may

help manage symptoms of benign prostatic hyperplasia (BPH), a non-cancerous enlargement of the prostate gland.

3. **Hormonal Balance:** Nettle root is believed to influence hormonal balance, particularly in men. It may have effects on certain hormones, including testosterone.

4. **Diuretic Effects:** Nettle root has diuretic properties, meaning it may help increase urine production. This can be beneficial for conditions involving fluid retention.

5. **Allergy Relief:** Although often associated with the stinging hairs on the leaves, nettle root is sometimes used for allergy relief. It is believed to have anti-allergenic properties and may help alleviate symptoms like sneezing and itching.

6. **Iron Content:** Nettle root contains iron and other minerals, making it a potential dietary supplement for individuals with iron-deficiency anemia.

7. **Hair and Skin Health:** Some herbalists and practitioners of traditional medicine recommend nettle root for promoting healthy hair and skin. It is believed to have nourishing effects on these tissues.

8. **Detoxification:** Nettle root is thought to have detoxifying properties, helping the body eliminate waste products and supporting overall cleansing.

9. **Adaptogenic Qualities:** Nettle root is sometimes classified as an adaptogen, a substance believed to help the body adapt to stress and promote balance.

It's important to note that while nettle root has a history of traditional use and some scientific support for certain benefits, individual responses may vary. Before using nettle root for medicinal purposes, especially for specific health conditions, individuals should consult with healthcare professionals. Additionally, sustainable harvesting practices are important to ensure the conservation of wild nettle populations.

OREGANO

Oregano (Origanum vulgare) is a flavorful herb belonging to the mint family, known for its robust taste and aromatic qualities. It's native to the Mediterranean region but is now cultivated and used worldwide in various culinary dishes, herbal remedies, and essential oils.

Here are key features and uses of oregano:

- **Appearance:** Oregano is a perennial herb with small, oval-shaped leaves that are dark green and aromatic. It produces clusters of tiny white, pink, or purple flowers. The leaves are often used fresh or dried for culinary and medicinal purposes.

- **Flavor and Aroma:** Oregano has a bold, slightly bitter taste with a warm and aromatic aroma. The flavor can range from mild to pungent, depending on the variety and growing conditions.

- **Culinary Uses:** Oregano is a staple herb in Mediterranean, Italian, and Mexican cuisines, adding depth and flavor to dishes. It's used to season sauces, soups, pizzas, pasta, roasted vegetables, meats (particularly lamb and poultry), salads, and marinades.

- **Medicinal Properties:** Oregano has been used in traditional medicine for its potential health benefits. It contains essential oils, such as carvacrol and thymol, known for their antibacterial, antifungal, and antioxidant properties.

- **Topical Use:** Oregano oil, when diluted, is sometimes used topically for its potential antimicrobial effects, aiding in skin conditions and supporting wound healing.

❧ **Preservative Properties:** Oregano's natural antibacterial properties have led to its use as a natural food preservative, helping to inhibit the growth of certain bacteria and fungi.

HEALTH BENEFITS:

1. **Antioxidant Properties:** Oregano is a rich source of antioxidants, including phenols and flavonoids, which help combat oxidative stress and neutralize free radicals. These antioxidants contribute to overall health and may lower the risk of chronic diseases.

2. **Antibacterial and Antifungal Effects:** Oregano contains compounds like carvacrol and thymol that exhibit potent antibacterial and antifungal properties. These properties make oregano useful in inhibiting the growth of certain harmful bacteria and fungi, potentially aiding in preventing infections.

3. **Anti-Inflammatory Benefits:** Compounds in oregano, particularly carvacrol and rosmarinic acid, possess anti-inflammatory properties. These properties may help reduce inflammation in the body, potentially benefiting conditions like arthritis.

4. **Respiratory Support:** Oregano's aromatic compounds may have mild expectorant properties, which could aid in respiratory health by helping to relieve coughs and congestion, promoting easier breathing.

5. **Immune System Support:** The antibacterial and antioxidant properties of oregano may contribute to its immune-boosting potential, helping the body fight off infections and supporting overall immune function.

6. **Potential Anti-Cancer Effects:** Some studies suggest that certain compounds in oregano may have anti-cancer properties, showing promise in inhibiting the growth of cancer cells. However, more research is needed to confirm and understand these effects fully.

7. **Heart Health:** Oregano's antioxidants and anti-inflammatory properties might contribute to cardiovascular health by potentially reducing inflammation and oxidative stress, factors associated with heart disease.

8. **Skin Health:** Oregano oil, when properly diluted, is used topically for its potential antimicrobial and soothing effects on skin conditions, such as acne or minor skin irritations.

9. **Digestive Aid:** Oregano's essential oils might stimulate digestive enzymes, promoting better nutrient absorption and aiding in the breakdown of fats, potentially benefiting overall digestive health.

While oregano offers potential health benefits, it's primarily used as a culinary herb. Consuming oregano in moderate amounts as part of a balanced diet is generally safe for most individuals. However, concentrated forms like essential oils should be used cautiously and properly diluted. Individuals with specific health conditions or allergies should consult a healthcare professional before using oregano for medicinal purposes.

PARSLEY

Parsley (Petroselinum crispum) is a versatile herb widely used in culinary dishes for its fresh flavor, as well as in traditional medicine for its potential health benefits. It belongs to the Apiaceae family and is known for its bright green leaves and a mild, slightly peppery taste.

Here are some key features and uses of parsley:

- **Appearance:** Parsley has vibrant green, flat or curly leaves, depending on the variety. It produces small, clustered flowers that are typically yellowish-green in color.

- **Flavor and Aroma:** Parsley has a fresh, slightly tangy flavor with a hint of bitterness and a mild peppery taste. The flavor can vary between the flat-leaf (Italian) parsley and the curly-leaf parsley.

- **Culinary Uses:** Parsley is a staple herb in various cuisines around the world, often used as a garnish or a flavor enhancer in salads, soups, stews, sauces, dressings, marinades, and as a seasoning for meats, fish, and vegetables. Flat-leaf parsley is favored for its stronger taste and is often used in cooking, while curly parsley is commonly used as a garnish.

HEALTH BENEFITS:

1. **Rich in Nutrients:** Parsley is a nutritional powerhouse, containing vitamins A, C, K, and folate, as well as minerals like calcium, potassium, and iron. These nutrients contribute to overall health and well-being.

2. **Antioxidant Properties:** Parsley contains flavonoids, carotenoids, and vitamin C, which act as antioxidants, neutralizing free radicals and reducing oxidative stress that can contribute to various chronic diseases.

3. **Supports Heart Health:** The antioxidants in parsley may help support heart health by reducing inflammation and oxidative stress, potentially lowering the risk of heart disease.

4. **Bone Health:** The high vitamin K content in parsley supports bone health by aiding in bone mineralization and density, potentially reducing the risk of osteoporosis.

5. **Immune Support:** Parsley's vitamin C content supports the immune system, aiding in fighting off infections and boosting overall immune function.

6. **Digestive Health:** Parsley contains compounds that may help improve digestion by stimulating the production of digestive enzymes, aiding in the breakdown of food and alleviating minor gastrointestinal discomforts.

7. **Diuretic Effects:** Parsley is believed to have mild diuretic properties, promoting the elimination of excess water and toxins from the body, potentially supporting kidney health.

8. **Anti-Inflammatory Effects:** Some compounds in parsley possess anti-inflammatory properties, potentially benefiting conditions associated with inflammation, such as arthritis or inflammatory disorders.

9. **Oral Health:** Chewing parsley leaves can help freshen breath due to its natural deodorizing properties and might have some antibacterial effects beneficial for oral health.

10. **Cancer-Fighting Potential:** Some studies suggest that the compounds in parsley, such as apigenin, might have anti-cancer properties, potentially inhibiting the growth of certain cancer cells. However, more research is needed to confirm these effects.

Parsley can be consumed fresh or dried and is commonly used in culinary preparations. Adding parsley to dishes or incorporating it into your diet can contribute to its potential health benefits. However, individuals with specific health conditions or allergies should consult a healthcare professional before using parsley for medicinal purposes.

PASSIFLORA (PASSIONFLOWER)

Passiflora, commonly known as passionflower, is a genus of flowering plants belonging to the Passifloraceae family. This diverse genus includes vines, shrubs, and herbaceous plants. Passionflowers are known for their unique and intricate flowers, often with a complex structure and vivid colors. Here are key features and uses of Passiflora:

- **Floral Characteristics:** The flowers of Passiflora are distinctive and showy, typically featuring a complex structure with radial or spiral arrangements of filaments, petals, and a central structure called the corona. The corona often has colorful and fringed filaments, adding to the flower's ornamental appeal.

- **Fruit:** Passionflowers produce fruit known as passion fruit. Depending on the species, the fruit may be round or oval, and the outer skin can be smooth or wrinkled. The pulp inside the fruit is juicy and may range in color from yellow to orange to purple, depending on the species.

- **Climbing Vines:** Many Passiflora species are climbing vines that use tendrils to support their growth. These vines are often cultivated for their ornamental value, and some are used as medicinal or culinary plants.

- **Culinary Use:** The fruit of certain Passiflora species, especially Passiflora edulis (purple passion fruit), is edible and commonly used in culinary applications. The fruit has a sweet and tangy flavor and is used in beverages, desserts, and as a fresh snack.

- **Medicinal Uses:** Some Passiflora species, particularly Passiflora incarnata (maypop), have been traditionally used in herbal medicine for their potential calming and sedative effects.

Passionflower supplements are sometimes used to promote relaxation and alleviate symptoms of stress and anxiety.

- **Traditional and Cultural Significance:** In various cultures, passionflowers hold symbolic and cultural significance. The unique floral structure has led to interpretations representing elements of the Christian faith, with parts of the flower associated with aspects of the crucifixion.

- **Biodiversity:** The Passiflora genus is vast and includes over 500 species. This diversity contributes to the biodiversity of the ecosystems where these plants are found, particularly in tropical and subtropical regions.

- **Butterfly Host Plants:** Passionflowers are known to be host plants for certain butterfly species, such as the Gulf Fritillary (Agraulis vanillae). Butterflies lay their eggs on the leaves of passionflower vines, and the caterpillars feed on the foliage.

- **Horticultural Interest:** Many Passiflora species and hybrids are cultivated for ornamental purposes. They are grown in gardens and landscapes for their attractive flowers, unique foliage, and, in some cases, for the production of edible fruit.

- **Adaptive Radiation:** The evolution of the Passiflora genus is an example of adaptive radiation, where different species have evolved to exploit various ecological niches. This has resulted in a wide range of forms and adaptations within the genus.

HEALTH BENEFITS

1. **Calming and Relaxation:** Passionflower has been traditionally used for its calming and sedative effects. It may help promote relaxation and alleviate symptoms of stress and anxiety.

2. **Improved Sleep:** Due to its calming properties, passionflower is sometimes used to improve sleep quality. It may be beneficial for individuals experiencing mild sleep disturbances or insomnia.

3. **Natural Sedative:** Passionflower has mild sedative properties, and herbal preparations are often used to induce relaxation without causing significant drowsiness.

4. **Anxiolytic Effects:** Some studies suggest that passionflower may have anxiolytic effects, helping to reduce feelings of anxiety. This is believed to be associated with certain compounds in the plant, such as flavonoids and alkaloids.

5. **Antispasmodic Properties:** Passionflower has been traditionally used as an antispasmodic, helping to relax muscles and relieve tension. It may be beneficial for conditions involving muscle spasms or cramps.

6. **Mood Enhancement:** Some people use passionflower for its potential mood-enhancing effects. It is believed to have a positive impact on overall emotional well-being.

7. **Support for Gastrointestinal Health:** Passionflower has been used in traditional medicine to support gastrointestinal health. It may help alleviate symptoms of indigestion and soothe the digestive tract.

8. **Anti-Inflammatory Effects:** Certain compounds found in passionflower, such as flavonoids, have been studied for their potential anti-inflammatory properties. This may contribute to the plant's traditional use for conditions involving inflammation.

9. **Cardiovascular Support:** Preliminary research suggests that passionflower may have cardiovascular benefits, including its potential to lower blood pressure. However, more research is needed to confirm these effects.

10. **Pain Relief:** Passionflower has been used traditionally for pain relief. It may help alleviate discomfort associated with various conditions, although further research is necessary to fully understand its analgesic properties.

11. **Menstrual Symptom Relief:** Some women use passionflower to alleviate symptoms associated with menstruation, such as cramps and anxiety.

12. **Antioxidant Activity:** Passionflower contains antioxidants, which may help neutralize free radicals in the body and protect cells from oxidative stress.

It's important to consult with healthcare professionals before using passionflower supplements, especially for individuals with pre-existing health conditions or those taking medications. Additionally, passionflower should not be used as a substitute for prescribed medications without proper medical guidance.

PEPPERMINT

Peppermint (Mentha × piperita) is a hybrid mint variety, a cross between watermint and spearmint, known for its refreshing aroma, cooling flavor, and various uses in culinary, medicinal, and aromatic applications.

Here are some key features and uses of peppermint:

- **Appearance:** Peppermint has serrated, bright green leaves with a distinct minty aroma. It produces small clusters of pink or purple flowers during its blooming season.

- **Flavor and Aroma:** Peppermint has a strong, refreshing, and cooling flavor with a distinct menthol taste. Its aroma is refreshing and minty, often associated with a cooling sensation.

- **Culinary Uses:** Peppermint is widely used in culinary applications. It's a popular flavoring agent in teas, beverages (like peppermint tea or mojitos), candies, desserts, ice creams, and savory dishes. It adds a refreshing and minty taste to various recipes.

- **Medicinal Properties:** Peppermint has been used in traditional medicine for its potential health benefits. It contains essential oils, primarily menthol, which contribute to its medicinal properties.

- **Aromatherapy:** Peppermint's invigorating scent is used in aromatherapy to promote alertness, mental clarity, and relaxation. Peppermint oil is often diffused for its refreshing aroma.

HEALTH BENEFITS:

1. **Digestive Health:** Peppermint is well-known for its digestive properties. It may help alleviate symptoms of indigestion, gas, bloating, and stomach discomfort by relaxing the muscles in the digestive tract and promoting the flow of bile.

2. **Relief from Irritable Bowel Syndrome (IBS):** Peppermint oil capsules or tea have been studied for their potential to alleviate symptoms of IBS, such as abdominal pain, bloating, and altered bowel movements, providing relief for some individuals.

3. **Respiratory Support:** Menthol, a compound found in peppermint, acts as a natural decongestant. Peppermint tea or inhaling peppermint oil vapors may help alleviate nasal congestion, soothe sore throats, and ease coughs by promoting easier breathing.

4. **Pain Relief:** Topical application of diluted peppermint oil may provide relief from headaches, migraines, muscle aches, and minor pains due to its cooling and analgesic effects.

5. **Antibacterial and Antifungal Effects:** Peppermint's essential oils, particularly menthol, possess potential antibacterial and antifungal properties, which may help inhibit the growth of certain bacteria and fungi.

6. **Mental Clarity and Alertness:** Peppermint's invigorating scent is used in aromatherapy to promote mental clarity, alertness, and relaxation. Inhaling peppermint oil vapors might improve focus and increase alertness.

7. **Oral Health:** Peppermint's antimicrobial properties make it a common ingredient in oral care products like toothpaste and mouthwash. It can help freshen breath and inhibit bacterial growth in the mouth.

8. **Anti-Inflammatory Effects:** Peppermint contains antioxidants and compounds with potential anti-inflammatory properties, which

may help reduce inflammation in the body, benefiting conditions like arthritis or inflammatory disorders.

9. **Stress Relief:** Peppermint's soothing aroma might have calming effects, reducing stress, and promoting relaxation when used in aromatherapy or through inhalation.

10. **Potential Skin Benefits:** Peppermint oil, when diluted, is sometimes used topically for its cooling sensation and potential benefits for soothing skin irritation, itchiness, or minor rashes.

While peppermint offers potential health benefits, it's important to use it in appropriate forms and amounts. Concentrated forms like essential oils should be properly diluted, and individuals with specific health conditions or allergies should consult a healthcare professional before using peppermint for medicinal purposes.

PRICKLY PEAR CACTUS

Prickly pear cactus refers to several species of cacti belonging to the Opuntia genus, and they are commonly found in arid and semi-arid regions of the Americas. These cacti are characterized by their flattened, pad-like stems, often covered with sharp spines or glochids. Here are key features and characteristics of the prickly pear cactus:

- **Botanical Characteristics:**
  - **Pads:** The stems of the prickly pear cactus are modified into flattened, paddle-shaped structures known as pads or cladodes. These pads can vary in size, shape, and color, depending on the species.
  - **Spines and Glochids:** Prickly pear cacti are armed with spines and glochids. Spines are larger, needle-like structures that can cause injury, while glochids are tiny, hair-like structures found in clusters on the pads. Glochids are barbed and easily detach, causing irritation upon contact.

- **Flowers:**
  - **Blossoms:** Prickly pear cacti produce vibrant, usually large and showy flowers that bloom in a range of colors, including yellow, orange, pink, and red.
  - **Blooming Season:** The flowering season varies among species, but many prickly pear cacti bloom in spring and early summer.

- **Fruits:**

- **Edible Fruit:** The fruit of the prickly pear cactus is commonly known as a "pear" or "tuna." It is fleshy, sweet, and edible. The color of the fruit can range from green to yellow, orange, or red, depending on the species.

- **Seeds:** The seeds of the prickly pear fruit are embedded in the flesh and are generally hard.

Ecological Adaptations:

- **Drought Tolerance:** Prickly pear cacti are well-adapted to arid environments and can withstand prolonged periods of drought.

- **Water Storage:** The stems of the prickly pear cactus are modified to store water, allowing the plant to survive in regions with limited water availability.

Culinary Uses:

- **Edible Pads:** The young pads (nopales) of some prickly pear cactus species are edible and are used in various culinary dishes. They are often cooked and added to salads, soups, or served as a side dish.

- **Edible Fruit:** The ripe fruit of the prickly pear cactus is also edible and can be eaten fresh or used in juices, jams, and desserts.

Landscaping and Ornamental Use:

- **Garden Plant:** Certain species of prickly pear cactus are cultivated for landscaping purposes. They are valued for their unique appearance, drought tolerance, and low maintenance.

Cultural and Symbolic Significance:

- **Symbolism:** In some cultures, the prickly pear cactus symbolizes endurance, strength, and resilience, given its ability to thrive in harsh and challenging environments.

HEALTH BENEFITS

1. **Rich in Nutrients:**

   - Prickly pear pads are a good source of vitamins, including vitamin C and various B vitamins.

   - The fruit of the prickly pear is rich in antioxidants, including vitamin C and carotenoids.

2. **Antioxidant Properties:** The antioxidants present in prickly pear, such as flavonoids and polyphenols, may help neutralize free radicals and protect cells from oxidative stress.

3. **Anti-Inflammatory Effects:** Some studies suggest that compounds in prickly pear may have anti-inflammatory properties, potentially contributing to the alleviation of inflammation in the body.

4. **Blood Sugar Control:**

   - Prickly pear may have hypoglycemic effects, helping to regulate blood sugar levels. This makes it of interest in the management of diabetes.

   - Certain compounds in prickly pear may slow the absorption of sugar in the digestive tract.

5. **Cholesterol Regulation:** Some research indicates that prickly pear may have cholesterol-lowering effects. It may help reduce levels of LDL cholesterol (the "bad" cholesterol) in the blood.

6. **Gastrointestinal Health:**

  - Prickly pear has been traditionally used to support digestive health. The mucilage in the pads may help soothe the digestive tract.

  - The fiber content of prickly pear may contribute to regular bowel movements and overall digestive well-being.

7. **Hydration:** The water content in prickly pear fruit contributes to hydration, making it a refreshing and hydrating option, especially in arid climates.

8. **Weight Management:** The fiber content in prickly pear may contribute to a feeling of fullness, potentially aiding in weight management.

9. **Anti-Infection Properties:** Certain compounds in prickly pear have been studied for their potential antimicrobial and antiviral properties.

10. **Liver Health:** Some studies suggest that prickly pear may have hepatoprotective effects, supporting liver health and protecting against liver damage.

11. **Skin Health:** The antioxidants in prickly pear may contribute to skin health by neutralizing free radicals that can lead to premature aging.

12. **Electrolyte Balance:** The potassium content in prickly pear may contribute to electrolyte balance in the body, supporting proper muscle and nerve function.

It's essential to consume prickly pear cactus in moderation, and individuals with certain health conditions, such as kidney issues or allergies, should consult with healthcare professionals before incorporating it into their diet. Additionally, proper identification and preparation of the plant parts are crucial to avoid potential allergic reactions or ingestion of spines.

RED CLOVER

Red clover (Trifolium pratense) is a flowering plant belonging to the legume family Fabaceae. It's a perennial herbaceous plant recognized for its distinctive globe-shaped red to purple flower heads and trifoliate (three-lobed) leaves.

Here are some key features and uses of red clover:

- **Appearance:** Red clover grows upright, with stems bearing clusters of small, reddish-pink flowers that form globe-shaped heads. The leaves are trifoliate, with three leaflets.

- **Habitat:** It's commonly found in meadows, fields, and grassy areas, often used as forage for livestock due to its nutritional value.

- **Culinary Uses:** Red clover is not a primary culinary herb but has been used historically in some cultures as a foraged edible green. It's occasionally added to salads or used as a garnish, although it's primarily valued for its potential medicinal properties rather than its culinary uses.

- **Medicinal Uses:** Red clover has been used in traditional herbal medicine for various purposes. It contains isoflavones, specifically biochanin A and formononetin, which are phytoestrogens believed to mimic the effects of estrogen in the body.

- **Forage and Soil Improvement:** Apart from its medicinal uses, red clover is also utilized as a forage crop for livestock and as a cover crop in agriculture to improve soil fertility due to its ability to fix nitrogen.

1. **Menopausal Symptom Relief:** Red clover is often used to alleviate menopausal symptoms such as hot flashes, night sweats, mood swings, and vaginal dryness. Its phytoestrogens may help mimic the effects of estrogen, potentially reducing the severity of these symptoms.

2. **Bone Health:** Phytoestrogens in red clover might support bone density and health, potentially reducing the risk of osteoporosis, a condition characterized by reduced bone mineral density and an increased risk of fractures.

3. **Cardiovascular Health:** Some studies suggest that red clover's isoflavones may contribute to heart health by potentially improving blood flow, reducing arterial stiffness, and modestly lowering LDL ("bad") cholesterol levels. These effects might help in reducing the risk of heart disease.

4. **Skin Health:** Red clover extracts or creams are sometimes used for skin conditions like eczema and psoriasis due to their potential anti-inflammatory properties, offering relief from itching and irritation.

5. **Antioxidant Effects:** Red clover contains antioxidants that help combat free radicals, reducing oxidative stress and potentially lowering the risk of chronic diseases associated with oxidative damage.

6. **Respiratory Support:** In traditional medicine, red clover has been used to ease coughs and soothe minor respiratory discomforts, although scientific evidence supporting this is limited.

7. **Women's Health:** Red clover supplements are occasionally used by women for breast health, although more research is needed to establish its effectiveness in this regard.

8. **Possible Cancer Prevention:** Some studies suggest that the isoflavones in red clover might have a role in reducing the risk of certain cancers, particularly hormone-related cancers like breast and prostate cancer. However, research in this area is ongoing and inconclusive.

It's crucial to consult with a healthcare professional before using red clover supplements, especially for individuals with hormone-related conditions, pregnant individuals, or those on medications, as it may interact with certain drugs or have contraindications. Additionally, relying solely on herbal remedies like red clover for serious health conditions should be done under proper medical guidance.

REISHI MUSHROOMS

Reishi mushroom, scientifically known as Ganoderma lucidum, is a species of mushroom that has been used for centuries in traditional medicine, particularly in East Asia. Also known as Lingzhi in China and Mannentake in Japan, Reishi is renowned for its potential health benefits. Here are key features and characteristics of the Reishi mushroom:

- **Physical Appearance:**

  - The Reishi mushroom has a distinctive appearance with a shiny, varnished cap that is typically kidney-shaped or fan-shaped. The cap surface can range in color from red to orange, black, or a combination of these hues.

  - The undersides of the cap have a white, porous surface.

- **Habitat:** Reishi mushrooms are typically found growing on decaying hardwood trees, especially on stumps or logs. They have a preference for mature hardwood forests.

- **Medicinal History:** Reishi has a long history of use in traditional Chinese medicine, where it is considered one of the most revered mushrooms for promoting health and longevity.

  - It has been referred to as the "Mushroom of Immortality" and the "Herb of Spiritual Potency."

- **Bioactive Compounds:** Reishi mushrooms contain various bioactive compounds, including triterpenoids, polysaccharides, ganoderic acids, and other antioxidants. These compounds are believed to contribute to the mushroom's potential health benefits.

HEALTH BENEFITS

1. **Adaptogenic Properties:** Reishi is classified as an adaptogen, which means it may help the body adapt to stress and promote balance in various physiological functions.

2. **Immune System Support:** Compounds in Reishi, particularly beta-glucans, are believed to modulate and enhance the activity of immune cells, potentially supporting the body's defense against infections and diseases.

3. **Anti-Inflammatory Effects:** Reishi mushrooms may have anti-inflammatory properties, which could be beneficial for conditions involving inflammation.

4. **Cardiovascular Health:** Some research suggests that Reishi may have positive effects on cardiovascular health by helping to regulate blood pressure and cholesterol levels.

5. **Potential Anticancer Effects:** Studies have explored the potential anticancer properties of Reishi mushrooms. Some compounds in Reishi may exhibit antitumor effects, although more research is needed in this area.

6. **Liver Health:** Reishi has been traditionally used to support liver health, and some studies suggest potential hepatoprotective effects.

7. **Stress Reduction:** Reishi's adaptogenic properties may contribute to stress reduction and improved mental well-being.

It's important to note that while Reishi mushroom has a long history of traditional use and some scientific support for certain health benefits, individual responses may vary. Before incorporating Reishi supplements into one's routine, consultation with healthcare professionals is advisable, especially for individuals with pre-existing health conditions or those taking medications.

RHAPONTICUM (MARAL ROOT)

Rhaponticum, commonly referred to as Rhaponticum carthamoides or Maral root, is a perennial herbaceous plant native to Siberia and parts of Central Asia. It is a member of the Asteraceae family and has been traditionally used in traditional medicine in certain regions. Here are key features and characteristics of Rhaponticum:

- **Botanical Characteristics:**

  - Rhaponticum carthamoides is a herbaceous plant with a thick, fleshy root that is often the part of the plant used for medicinal purposes.

  - The plant typically grows to a height of about 30 to 68 centimeters.

- **Leaves and Flowers:**

  - The leaves are lance-shaped and may have serrated edges.

  - Rhaponticum produces yellow flowers that are arranged in a cluster, typical of plants in the Asteraceae family.

- **Common Names:** Besides Rhaponticum carthamoides, this plant is known by various common names, including Maral root, Russian Leuzea, and Rhaponticum.

- **Habitat:** Rhaponticum is native to the Altai Mountains in Siberia and can be found in other parts of Central Asia. It often grows in meadows, rocky slopes, and forested areas.

- **Traditional Uses:** The root of Rhaponticum carthamoides has been used in traditional medicine in certain cultures for various purposes, including as an adaptogen and for its potential to enhance physical performance.

- **Endangered Status:** In some regions, Rhaponticum carthamoides has faced habitat loss and overharvesting, leading to concerns about its status in the wild. Conservation efforts are underway to protect and sustainably manage populations.

- **Supplements and Extracts:** Rhaponticum carthamoides is available in various forms, including supplements and extracts, for those interested in its potential health benefits.

HEALTH BENEFITS

1. **Adaptogenic Properties:** Like many other plants in the adaptogen category, Rhaponticum is believed to have properties that help the body adapt to stress and promote overall balance.

2. **Potential for Physical Performance:** In traditional usage and some studies, Rhaponticum carthamoides has been associated with potential benefits for physical performance. It is believed to have tonic effects that may enhance endurance and stamina.

3. **Phytochemical Composition:** Rhaponticum contains various bioactive compounds, including ecdysteroids, flavonoids, polyacetylenes, and essential oils. Ecdysteroids are a group of compounds that have been of particular interest due to their potential effects on muscle protein synthesis and physical performance.

4. **Research and Studies:** While traditional usage suggests certain benefits, scientific research on Rhaponticum carthamoides is ongoing, and more studies are needed to fully understand its effects and mechanisms of action.

It's important to approach the use of Rhaponticum carthamoides or its extracts with caution. Individuals considering its supplementation should consult with healthcare professionals, especially if they have pre-existing health conditions or are taking medications. Additionally, sustainable harvesting practices and conservation efforts are crucial to ensure the protection of this plant species in its natural habitat.

ROSEMARY

Rosemary (Rosmarinus officinalis) is an aromatic evergreen herb known for its fragrant needle-like leaves and various culinary, medicinal, and aromatic uses. It belongs to the mint family, Lamiaceae, and is native to the Mediterranean region.

Here are key features and uses of rosemary:

- **Appearance:** Rosemary is an evergreen shrub with needle-like leaves that are dark green on top and silvery-white underneath. It produces small, blue, purple, or white flowers, and its leaves are highly aromatic.

- **Flavor and Aroma:** Rosemary has a robust, pine-like aroma with a slightly bitter, earthy flavor. It's used to add a distinctive taste and aroma to various dishes.

- **Culinary Uses:** Rosemary is a popular culinary herb used in Mediterranean cuisine. It's commonly used to flavor roasted meats (especially lamb and chicken), vegetables, soups, stews, marinades, bread, and savory baked goods. It pairs well with garlic, olive oil, and citrus flavors.

- **Medicinal Properties:** Rosemary has been used in traditional medicine for its potential health benefits. It contains various compounds, including antioxidants, essential oils (like cineole and camphor), and rosmarinic acid.

- **Aromatherapy:** The invigorating scent of rosemary is used in aromatherapy to promote relaxation, mental clarity, and alertness. Rosemary oil is often diffused for its aromatic benefits.

1. **Liver Health:** Rosemary contains compounds that might support liver health by promoting detoxification processes and potentially protecting the liver from damage caused by toxins.

2. **Anti-Diabetic Effects:** Some research suggests that rosemary extracts may help regulate blood sugar levels and improve insulin sensitivity, potentially offering benefits for individuals with diabetes.

3. **Anti-Cancer Properties:** Certain compounds in rosemary, such as rosmarinic acid and carnosol, have shown potential anti-cancer effects in laboratory studies, exhibiting properties that may inhibit the growth of cancer cells.

4. **Eye Health:** Rosemary contains nutrients like vitamin A, which is essential for eye health. It might contribute to maintaining good vision and reducing the risk of age-related eye conditions.

5. **Immune System Support:** The antioxidants in rosemary may contribute to supporting the immune system by neutralizing free radicals and promoting overall immune function.

6. **Antimicrobial Properties:** Rosemary's essential oils have demonstrated antimicrobial activity against certain bacteria and fungi, suggesting potential benefits in preventing certain infections.

7. **Improved Circulation:** Compounds in rosemary may help improve circulation by dilating blood vessels, potentially promoting better blood flow throughout the body.

8. **Stress Reduction:** Inhalation of rosemary oil or exposure to its aroma through aromatherapy may help reduce stress levels and promote relaxation due to its soothing and invigorating scent.

While these health benefits are associated with rosemary, more research is needed to fully understand its effects on various health conditions. Using rosemary in culinary amounts is generally safe for most people, but concentrated forms or supplements should be used cautiously. Individuals with specific health concerns or those taking medications should consult a healthcare professional before using rosemary for medicinal purposes.

SAFFRON

Saffron (Crocus sativus) is a highly valued and aromatic spice derived from the flower of the saffron crocus plant. Here are key features and characteristics of saffron:

- **Botanical Characteristics:** Saffron crocus is a small, perennial plant belonging to the Iridaceae family. It has slender, grass-like leaves and purple flowers with a central three-pronged stigma.

- **Saffron Threads:** The most valuable part of the saffron flower is the stigma, a thread-like structure in the center. These threads, known as saffron strands or saffron threads, are hand-harvested and dried to produce the spice.

- **Color and Flavor:** Saffron imparts a vivid golden-yellow to orange-red color to dishes. It is known for its distinctive and complex flavor profile, which includes floral, honey, and hay-like notes. The taste is subtle and can be slightly bitter.

- **Aroma:** Saffron has a strong, aromatic fragrance that intensifies when the threads are steeped or used in cooking. The aroma is a key factor in its culinary appeal.

- **Culinary Uses:**

  - Saffron is a prized spice in various cuisines worldwide, particularly in Middle Eastern, Mediterranean, Indian, and Spanish dishes.

  - It is used to flavor and color a wide range of dishes, including rice, stews, soups, and desserts.

- **Culinary Applications:**

- Saffron is often used in the preparation of paella, biryani, risotto, and various sweet treats like saffron-infused pastries and ice creams.

  - It is a key ingredient in traditional dishes like Iranian saffron rice and Spanish saffron-infused sauces.

- **Expensive and Labor-Intensive:** Saffron is one of the most expensive spices in the world due to the labor-intensive process of harvesting. Each saffron crocus flower yields only a small number of threads.

- **Cultivation Regions:** Saffron is primarily cultivated in regions with a Mediterranean climate, including Iran, India, Spain, Greece, and parts of the Middle East.

- **Harvesting:** Saffron threads are harvested during the blooming season in autumn. The delicate threads are carefully plucked from the flowers by hand.

- **Saffron Production:** The labor-intensive harvesting process and the need for a large number of flowers to produce a small amount of saffron contribute to its high cost.

- **Symbolism:** Saffron has cultural and symbolic significance in various traditions. It is associated with luxury, royalty, and auspicious occasions.

HEALTH BENEFITS

1. **Antioxidant Properties:** Saffron is rich in antioxidants, such as crocin, crocetin, and safranal. These compounds help neutralize free radicals in the body, reducing oxidative stress.

2. **Anti-Inflammatory Effects:** Some studies suggest that saffron may possess anti-inflammatory properties, which could be beneficial in managing inflammatory conditions.

3. **Mood Enhancement:** Saffron has been studied for its potential antidepressant effects. Compounds in saffron may influence neurotransmitters like serotonin, contributing to improved mood.

4. **Cognitive Function:** Preliminary research indicates that saffron may have neuroprotective effects, potentially enhancing cognitive function and protecting against age-related decline.

5. **Improved Sleep:** Saffron has been investigated for its potential to improve sleep quality. Compounds like crocin may have a relaxing effect on the central nervous system.

6. **Anti-Cancer Properties:** Some studies suggest that saffron may have anti-cancer properties, inhibiting the growth of cancer cells and inducing apoptosis (programmed cell death).

7. **Cardiovascular Health:** Saffron may contribute to cardiovascular health by helping regulate blood pressure and improving lipid profiles. Antioxidants in saffron may protect against heart disease.

8. **Anti-Diabetic Effects:** Research has explored the potential of saffron in managing diabetes. It may help lower blood sugar levels and improve insulin sensitivity.

9. **Menstrual Health:** Saffron has been traditionally used to alleviate symptoms of premenstrual syndrome (PMS) and menstrual discomfort. It may have a regulatory effect on hormones.

10. **Aphrodisiac Properties:** Saffron has a historical reputation as an aphrodisiac. Some studies suggest that it may have positive effects on sexual function.

11. **Eye Health:** Compounds like crocin may have protective effects on the retina, potentially benefiting eye health.

12. **Anti-Anxiety Effects:** Saffron has been studied for its potential anxiolytic effects, offering a calming influence and helping to reduce symptoms of anxiety.

13. **Weight Management:** Some research indicates that saffron may help in weight management by reducing appetite and promoting a feeling of fullness.

It's important to note that while saffron shows promise in these areas, more extensive and rigorous research is needed to establish its efficacy and safety for specific health conditions. Additionally, individual responses may vary, and saffron supplements should be used with caution, especially in therapeutic doses. Consulting with healthcare professionals is advisable, especially for those with existing health conditions or individuals taking medications.

SAGE

Sage (Salvia officinalis) is an aromatic herb known for its distinct flavor, fragrance, and various culinary, medicinal, and ceremonial uses. It belongs to the mint family, Lamiaceae, and is native to the Mediterranean region.

Here are key features and uses of sage:

- **Appearance:** Sage is an evergreen perennial plant with woody stems, grayish-green leaves that are velvety and lance-shaped, and it produces small, purple, blue, or white flowers.

- **Flavor and Aroma:** Sage has a robust, earthy flavor with a slightly bitter and warm taste. It emits a strong, aromatic fragrance when its leaves are crushed or rubbed.

- **Culinary Uses:** Sage is a popular culinary herb used in various cuisines worldwide, especially in Mediterranean dishes. It's used to flavor meats (such as pork, poultry, and sausages), stuffings, soups, stews, sauces, pasta, and savory baked goods. It pairs well with fatty or rich foods.

- **Medicinal Properties:** Sage has been used in traditional medicine for its potential health benefits. It contains various compounds, including rosmarinic acid, flavonoids, and essential oils like thujone.

HEALTH BENEFITS:

1. **Diabetes Management:** Some studies suggest that sage might help manage diabetes by potentially improving insulin sensitivity and reducing blood sugar levels, though more research is needed to confirm its efficacy.

2. **Skin Health:** Sage contains antioxidants and anti-inflammatory properties that may benefit skin health. It's sometimes used topically in skincare products or diluted in oils to soothe minor skin irritations and reduce inflammation.

3. **Antibacterial and Antiviral Effects:** Sage's essential oils have demonstrated antimicrobial properties against certain bacteria and viruses, suggesting potential benefits in preventing infections or supporting immune health.

4. **Mood Enhancement:** Inhalation of sage oil or exposure to its aroma through aromatherapy is believed to have mood-enhancing effects, promoting relaxation and potentially reducing anxiety and stress.

5. **Hair and Scalp Benefits:** Sage oil is sometimes used in hair care products or diluted in carrier oils to promote scalp health, stimulate hair growth, and reduce dandruff due to its antimicrobial properties.

6. **Improved Memory and Mental Clarity:** Some studies indicate that compounds in sage might support cognitive function, potentially enhancing memory and mental alertness, though more research is needed for conclusive evidence.

7. **Respiratory Support:** Sage's aromatic properties may have a soothing effect on the respiratory system. Inhaling steam with sage may provide relief from congestion and support respiratory health.

8. **Bone Health:** The presence of certain compounds in sage might support bone health by aiding in bone density and potentially

reducing the risk of osteoporosis. However, further research is required to confirm this effect.

Always use sage and its derivatives in appropriate amounts, and consult with a healthcare professional, especially if you have specific health concerns, are pregnant, or are taking medications, as sage may interact with certain medications or have contraindications for certain individuals.

SIBERIAN GINSENG

Siberian ginseng, scientifically known as Eleutherococcus senticosus, is a plant native to Eastern Asia, particularly Siberia, China, Japan, and Korea. Despite its name, Siberian ginseng is not botanically related to true ginseng (Panax ginseng) but shares some adaptogenic properties. Here are key features and characteristics of Siberian ginseng:

- **Botanical Characteristics:** Siberian ginseng is a deciduous shrub with compound leaves and small, clustered, greenish-yellow flowers. The plant reaches a height of about 2 to 3 meters.

- **Common Names:** Besides Siberian ginseng, Eleutherococcus senticosus is also known by various names, including eleuthero and ciwujia.

- **Adaptogenic Properties:** Siberian ginseng is classified as an adaptogen, a category of herbs believed to help the body adapt to stress and restore balance. It is thought to support the body's resistance to physical, chemical, and biological stressors.

- **Traditional Uses:**In traditional Chinese medicine and Russian folk medicine, Siberian ginseng has been used for centuries to enhance stamina, promote overall well-being, and address conditions related to stress and fatigue.

- **Active Compounds:** Siberian ginseng contains various bioactive compounds, including eleutherosides, polysaccharides, triterpenoids, and flavonoids. These compounds are believed to contribute to its adaptogenic and immune-modulating effects.

HEALTH BENEFITS

1. **Immune System Support:** Siberian ginseng is thought to modulate the immune system, potentially enhancing immune function and promoting overall immune health.

2. **Physical Performance and Endurance:** Some studies suggest that Siberian ginseng may have benefits for physical performance and endurance. It is believed to help the body adapt to stressors during exercise.

3. **Cognitive Function:** Siberian ginseng has been investigated for its potential effects on cognitive function. Some studies suggest it may have neuroprotective properties and may help improve mental alertness and concentration.

4. **Stress Reduction:** As an adaptogen, Siberian ginseng is believed to have stress-reducing effects. It may help the body cope with stress and alleviate symptoms of stress and fatigue.

5. **Antioxidant Properties:** Siberian ginseng exhibits antioxidant activity, helping to neutralize free radicals in the body and protect cells from oxidative stress.

6. **Anti-Inflammatory Effects:** Some studies suggest that Siberian ginseng may have anti-inflammatory properties, potentially contributing to its overall health benefits.

7. **Cardiovascular Health:** Siberian ginseng has been studied for its potential cardiovascular benefits, including its effects on blood pressure and cholesterol levels.

8. **Adrenal Support:** Siberian ginseng is believed to support adrenal function, helping the body better cope with stress and fatigue.

9. **Regulatory Effects on Hormones:** It is suggested that Siberian ginseng may have regulatory effects on certain hormones, potentially benefiting conditions related to hormonal imbalances.

It's important to note that while Siberian ginseng is generally considered safe for most people when used appropriately, individual responses may vary. As with any herbal supplement, it's advisable to consult with healthcare professionals before incorporating Siberian ginseng into one's routine, especially for individuals with pre-existing health conditions or those taking medications.

SLIPPERY ELM

Slippery elm (Ulmus rubra) is a deciduous tree native to North America, particularly the eastern and central regions. The inner bark of the slippery elm tree has been traditionally used for its medicinal properties, and it has a long history of use by Native American tribes. Here are key features and characteristics of slippery elm:

- **Botanical Characteristics:** Slippery elm is a medium to large-sized tree that can reach heights of up to 80 feet. It has rough, reddish-brown bark, and its leaves are ovate with serrated edges.

- **Inner Bark:** The inner bark of the slippery elm tree is the part traditionally used for medicinal purposes. It has a mucilaginous texture when mixed with water, which gives it a slippery and slimy consistency.

- **Traditional Uses:** Native American tribes have historically used slippery elm for various medicinal purposes, including as a demulcent to soothe the throat and gastrointestinal tract.

- **Wildlife Value:** Apart from its historical and medicinal uses, slippery elm also holds value for wildlife. The tree provides food for various animals, and its wood is used by birds for nesting.

- **Conservation Status:** Slippery elm has faced challenges, including Dutch elm disease, which has affected many elm species. Conservation efforts are in place to protect and preserve this native tree.

HEALTH BENEFITS

1. **Demulcent Properties:** Slippery elm is known for its demulcent or mucilaginous properties. When the inner bark is mixed with water, it forms a gel-like substance that can provide a soothing coating to irritated tissues.

2. **Gastrointestinal Support:** Slippery elm has been traditionally used to support gastrointestinal health. It may help soothe irritation in the stomach and intestines, making it useful for conditions such as heartburn, indigestion, and ulcers.

3. **Throat Soother:** Due to its mucilaginous nature, slippery elm is often used to soothe sore throats and alleviate coughs. It can be consumed as a tea or lozenge.

4. **Respiratory Support:** Slippery elm has been used to provide relief for respiratory conditions such as bronchitis and coughs. It is believed to help soothe irritated mucous membranes.

5. **Skin Health:** External preparations containing slippery elm, such as salves or poultices, have been used topically to soothe skin irritations, burns, and wounds.

6. **Nutrient Content:** Slippery elm bark contains various nutrients, including tannins, mucilage, calcium, and other trace minerals.

7. **Historical Use by Soldiers:** During the American Revolution, soldiers reportedly used slippery elm as a makeshift food source during times of scarcity. The inner bark was dried and ground into a powder, which was then mixed with water.

While slippery elm has a history of traditional use and is generally considered safe, it's important to consult with healthcare professionals before using it for medicinal purposes, especially if an individual has underlying health conditions or is taking medications. Additionally, the conservation of native trees like slippery elm is crucial for maintaining biodiversity and ecosystem health.

SOURSOP

Soursop, also known as Graviola or Annona muricata, is a tropical fruit originating from the Caribbean, Central America, and parts of South America. It belongs to the Annonaceae family and is recognized for its prickly green exterior and soft, fibrous, white flesh inside. The fruit is renowned for its unique flavor profile, combining elements of strawberry, pineapple, and citrus notes.

Here are key features and uses of soursop:

- **Appearance:** Soursop is a spiky, heart-shaped fruit that can grow quite large, typically ranging from 5 to 12 inches in length and weighing several pounds. Its green, thorny exterior encases the soft, white, juicy flesh.

- **Flavor and Texture:** The flesh of the soursop fruit is creamy and fibrous, with a distinct, tropical flavor that's a blend of tangy and sweet, often likened to a mix of strawberry, pineapple, and citrus fruits.

- **Culinary Uses:** Soursop is primarily consumed fresh as a fruit or blended into beverages like juices, smoothies, and shakes. It's occasionally used in desserts, ice creams, sorbets, or incorporated into savory dishes in some cuisines.

- **Nutritional Profile:** Soursop is rich in vitamins and minerals, particularly vitamin C, vitamin B6, potassium, thiamine, and fiber. It's relatively low in calories but offers essential nutrients.

- **Medicinal Uses:** Traditional medicine in various cultures has used different parts of the soursop plant (leaves, bark, and fruit) for their potential medicinal properties. It's been associated with potential anti-inflammatory, antioxidant, and antimicrobial effects.

- **Antioxidant Properties:** Soursop contains antioxidants like flavonoids and polyphenols, which help neutralize free radicals, reducing oxidative stress and potentially lowering the risk of certain diseases.

- **Potential Health Benefits:** While further research is ongoing, some studies suggest that soursop may have properties that support immune function, digestive health, and may have anticancer properties. However, these claims require further scientific investigation.

- **Herbal Tea:** Soursop leaves are sometimes used to prepare herbal teas believed to offer health benefits. The tea is thought to have calming effects and potential digestive benefits.

- **Pest Control:** In some regions, soursop extracts are used in agriculture as a natural pest control measure against certain insects.

HEALTH BENEFITS:

1. **Digestive Health:** Soursop is rich in dietary fiber, which supports digestive health by promoting regular bowel movements, preventing constipation, and aiding in overall gastrointestinal function.

2. **Skin Health:** Some cultures use soursop extracts or pulp topically to promote skin health. It's believed to possess properties that may soothe skin irritations, reduce inflammation, and support wound healing.

3. **Potential Anti-Parasitic Effects:** Soursop has been traditionally used in some cultures as a natural remedy against parasites, particularly intestinal worms. Some studies suggest that soursop extracts might possess anti-parasitic properties.

4. **Anti-Inflammatory Properties:** Compounds found in soursop, such as acetogenins and antioxidants, exhibit potential anti-inflammatory effects. These properties may help reduce inflammation in the body and alleviate related conditions.

5. **Liver Health:** Soursop may have hepatoprotective properties, potentially supporting liver health by protecting liver cells from damage caused by toxins or oxidative stress.

6. **Potential Anti-Diabetic Effects:** Some preliminary studies suggest that certain compounds in soursop may help regulate blood sugar levels and improve insulin sensitivity, though further research is needed to confirm these effects.

7. **Cardiovascular Support:** Soursop contains potassium, which is beneficial for heart health. Adequate potassium intake helps regulate blood pressure and supports overall cardiovascular function.

8. **Stress Reduction:** The calming properties associated with soursop, particularly from consuming soursop tea, may help reduce stress levels and promote relaxation.

9. **Eye Health:** Soursop is a source of antioxidants like vitamin C and other compounds that may contribute to maintaining good vision and supporting overall eye health.

Remember, while soursop is a nutritious fruit with potential health benefits, consuming it in moderation as part of a balanced diet is advisable. Consulting a healthcare professional before using soursop for medicinal purposes is recommended, especially if you have existing health conditions or are taking medications.

St. John's Wort (Hypericum perforatum) is a flowering plant with yellow, star-shaped flowers native to Europe, parts of Asia, and North Africa. It's recognized for its traditional medicinal uses and is often used as an herbal remedy for various health conditions.

Key features and uses of St. John's Wort:

- **Appearance:** St. John's Wort is a herbaceous plant that grows upright, typically reaching heights between 1 to 3 feet. It features clusters of bright yellow flowers with five petals and translucent dots, along with opposite, oblong leaves that appear perforated when held up to light.

- **Medicinal Uses:** St. John's Wort has a long history of use in traditional medicine, primarily for its potential antidepressant and mood-enhancing effects. It contains active compounds like hypericin, hyperforin, and flavonoids believed to influence neurotransmitters in the brain.

- **Mental Health:** It's commonly used as a natural remedy to alleviate symptoms of mild to moderate depression, anxiety, and mood disorders. Some research suggests that St. John's Wort may increase levels of serotonin, dopamine, and norepinephrine in the brain, contributing to its potential mood-stabilizing effects.

HEALTH BENEFITS:

1. **Potential Antiviral Effects:** St. John's Wort has shown some promise in laboratory studies for its antiviral properties. It might exhibit activity against certain viruses, potentially aiding in combating viral infections.

2. **Wound Healing:** When applied topically, St. John's Wort oil or extracts have been traditionally used to assist in wound healing. Its anti-inflammatory and antimicrobial properties may help soothe minor skin injuries and promote healing.

3. **Possible Anti-Anxiety Effects:** Beyond its known antidepressant properties, some individuals use St. John's Wort to alleviate symptoms of anxiety or stress. However, scientific evidence supporting its efficacy in treating anxiety is limited.

4. **Neuroprotective Potential:** Some research suggests that compounds found in St. John's Wort may have neuroprotective effects, potentially supporting brain health and protecting against certain neurodegenerative conditions. Further studies are necessary to confirm these effects.

5. **Management of Obsessive-Compulsive Disorder (OCD):** There's some anecdotal evidence suggesting that St. John's Wort might assist in managing symptoms of OCD, but clinical research is required to substantiate these claims.

6. **Skin Conditions:** St. John's Wort's anti-inflammatory and antibacterial properties have led to its use in managing certain skin conditions, such as eczema or psoriasis. It may help reduce inflammation and soothe irritated skin.

7. **Possible Anticancer Properties:** Some studies have indicated that certain components of St. John's Wort may possess anticancer properties, showing potential in inhibiting the growth of certain cancer cells. However, more research is needed in this area.

8. **Prevention of Neural Damage:** In animal studies, St. John's Wort
   has shown potential in preventing nerve damage caused by toxins.
   It may have protective effects on nerve tissues, although human
   studies are needed to confirm these effects.

As with any herbal supplement or remedy, it's crucial to consult with a
healthcare professional before using St. John's Wort, especially if you're
on medication, pregnant, nursing, or have underlying health conditions.
This helps ensure safety, avoid potential interactions, and determine
appropriate dosages.

TARRAGON

Tarragon (Artemisia dracunculus) is a perennial herb belonging to the Asteraceae family and is native to Eurasia. It's renowned for its distinctive aromatic leaves and is a common ingredient in various cuisines, particularly French and Mediterranean.

Key features and uses of tarragon:

- **Appearance:** Tarragon is an herbaceous plant that grows as a perennial with narrow, lance-shaped leaves that are dark green in color. It produces small, pale green or white flowers in summer.

- **Flavor and Aroma:** Tarragon has a unique flavor profile, characterized by a mild anise or licorice-like taste with slightly sweet and peppery undertones. Its aroma is herbaceous and reminiscent of anise.

- **Culinary Uses:** Tarragon is a popular culinary herb used to flavor a variety of dishes. It's particularly favored in French cuisine, where it's a key ingredient in fines herbes and béarnaise sauce. It pairs well with poultry, seafood, eggs, vegetables, and dressings. Tarragon vinegar and tarragon-infused oils are also common.

- **Medicinal Properties:** In traditional medicine, tarragon has been used for its potential health benefits, including as a digestive aid and to stimulate appetite. It contains certain compounds that might have mild antioxidant properties.

- **Aromatherapy:** The aromatic properties of tarragon oil or the herb itself have been used in aromatherapy to promote relaxation and calmness.

- **Herbal Tea:** Tarragon leaves are occasionally used to prepare herbal teas. The tea is believed to offer a mild, soothing effect and is sometimes used to alleviate minor symptoms of insomnia or anxiety.

- **Preservative Properties:** Tarragon's antimicrobial properties have led to its historical use as a preservative in food, particularly in pickling or fermenting processes.

HEALTH BENEFITS:

1. **Regulation of Blood Sugar:** Tarragon has been studied for its potential to regulate blood sugar levels. Some research suggests that certain compounds in tarragon might assist in controlling blood sugar spikes, potentially beneficial for individuals with diabetes or those managing blood sugar levels.

2. **Bone Health:** Tarragon contains minerals like calcium and magnesium, which are essential for maintaining strong and healthy bones. Regular consumption of foods rich in these minerals, including tarragon, may contribute to bone health.

3. **Support for Oral Health:** Tarragon's antimicrobial properties have been associated with promoting oral health. It may help in reducing oral bacteria, potentially contributing to improved overall oral hygiene and fresher breath.

4. **Menstrual Health:** In traditional medicine, tarragon has been used to alleviate symptoms related to menstruation, such as menstrual cramps or irregular periods. Some believe it might help regulate menstrual cycles, although scientific evidence is limited.

5. **Diuretic Properties:** Tarragon has diuretic properties that may promote increased urine production. This effect might assist in reducing water retention and supporting kidney function, aiding in the elimination of waste from the body.

6. **Respiratory Support:** In some cultures, tarragon has been used to support respiratory health. It's believed to have expectorant properties, potentially aiding in the clearance of mucus and soothing minor respiratory discomforts.

7. **Digestive Health:** Tarragon has been suggested to stimulate the production of digestive enzymes, aiding in the digestion of food. It may help alleviate digestive issues like bloating and gas.

While tarragon offers potential health benefits, more scientific research is needed to substantiate many of these claims. It's essential to consume tarragon as part of a balanced diet and consult a healthcare professional before using it medicinally, especially for individuals with specific health concerns, pregnant individuals, or those on medications, to avoid potential interactions or adverse effects.

THYME

Thyme (Thymus vulgaris) is an aromatic herb from the mint family, Lamiaceae, known for its small leaves, fragrant aroma, and culinary and medicinal uses. It's native to the Mediterranean region but is now cultivated and used worldwide.

Key features and uses of thyme:

- **Appearance:** Thyme is a low-growing, perennial herb with tiny, elliptical leaves that are typically green-gray in color. It produces small, pale pink to lilac flowers in clusters during the summer.

- **Flavor and Aroma:** Thyme has a distinctive, earthy flavor with hints of mint and lemon. Its aroma is aromatic, herbaceous, and somewhat floral, making it a versatile herb in various cuisines.

- **Culinary Uses:** Thyme is a staple herb in Mediterranean and French cuisines, used to flavor a wide range of dishes. It pairs well with meats (especially poultry), vegetables, soups, stews, sauces, marinades, and stuffing. It's commonly used in dried form, but fresh thyme sprigs are also popular.

- **Medicinal Properties:** Thyme has been used in traditional medicine for its potential health benefits. It contains compounds like thymol and carvacrol, which possess antimicrobial and antioxidant properties.

- **Aromatherapy:** Thyme essential oil is used in aromatherapy for its calming and soothing effects. Its aroma is believed to promote relaxation and reduce stress.

- **Topical Uses:** Thyme oil or infusions have been used topically to address minor skin irritations, wounds, and insect bites due to its potential antiseptic properties.

Thyme is a versatile herb used in various forms, from dried leaves to essential oils, and is generally considered safe for culinary use. However, concentrated forms should be used cautiously and properly diluted. Individuals with specific health conditions or those taking medications should consult a healthcare professional before using thyme for medicinal purposes.

HEALTH BENEFITS:

1. **Boosting Immune Function:** Thyme contains vitamins, such as vitamin C, which contribute to immune system function. Its antimicrobial properties might also support overall immune health by combating certain infections.

2. **Potential Anti-Inflammatory Effects:** Compounds found in thyme, including rosmarinic acid and flavonoids, exhibit potential anti-inflammatory properties. Thyme extracts have shown promise in reducing inflammation, which may benefit conditions like arthritis.

3. **Cognitive Support:** Some research suggests that thyme might have cognitive benefits. Certain compounds in thyme have been studied for their potential to support brain health, memory, and cognitive function, though more research is needed for conclusive evidence.

4. **Antifungal Properties:** Thyme's active compounds, particularly thymol, have shown antifungal properties in some studies. Thyme

extracts may inhibit the growth of certain fungi, potentially helpful in addressing fungal infections.

5. **Support for Respiratory Health:** Thyme has expectorant properties that might aid in loosening phlegm and mucus, making it easier to expel, which can be beneficial in managing respiratory conditions like bronchitis or chest congestion.

6. **Heart Health:** Some studies suggest that thyme might have potential benefits for cardiovascular health. Compounds in thyme may help dilate blood vessels and improve blood flow, potentially aiding in blood pressure regulation.

7. **Antispasmodic Effects:** Thyme has been used traditionally as an antispasmodic agent to alleviate muscle spasms or cramps. Its relaxant properties might help ease muscular tension.

8. **Antiparasitic Properties:** Certain studies have explored the potential of thyme extracts to combat certain parasites. Thyme might possess properties that inhibit the growth of certain parasites, although more research is needed.

As with any herbal remedy or supplement, it's important to incorporate thyme into a balanced diet and lifestyle. Consulting with a healthcare professional is recommended, especially for individuals with specific health conditions, pregnant individuals, or those on medications, to ensure safe and appropriate usage of thyme for medicinal purposes.

TURMERIC

Turmeric (Curcuma longa) is a bright yellow-orange spice native to South Asia, commonly used in cooking and valued for its medicinal properties. It belongs to the ginger family, Zingiberaceae, and has been used for centuries in traditional medicine.

Key features and uses of turmeric:

- **Appearance:** Turmeric comes from the rhizomes of the turmeric plant. It's a vibrant yellow-orange spice that's ground into a fine powder. The fresh rhizome resembles ginger, with a bright orange interior.

- **Flavor and Aroma:** Turmeric has a warm, slightly bitter taste with a peppery and earthy flavor profile. Its aroma is mild and slightly reminiscent of orange and ginger.

- **Culinary Uses:** Turmeric is a staple in South Asian and Middle Eastern cuisines. It's a key ingredient in curry powders, providing both color and flavor to dishes. It's used in various recipes, including curries, soups, rice dishes, and marinades. It's also used to add color to foods like mustard and cheese.

- **Medicinal Properties:** Turmeric contains a bioactive compound called curcumin, which is responsible for many of its health benefits. Curcumin is a potent antioxidant and has anti-inflammatory properties.

HEALTH BENEFITS:

1. **Potential Anticancer Properties:** Curcumin, the active compound in turmeric, has been studied for its potential in cancer prevention and treatment. It's believed to interfere with the development, growth, and spread of cancer cells and might have potential as a complementary therapy, though more research is needed.

2. **Potential for Heart Health:** Some studies suggest that curcumin may have cardiovascular benefits, potentially improving the function of the endothelium (the lining of blood vessels) and contributing to heart health.

3. **Brain Health:** Curcumin's anti-inflammatory and antioxidant properties have sparked interest in its potential to support brain health and potentially reduce the risk of neurodegenerative diseases, although more research is needed.

4. **Wound Healing:** Turmeric has been used topically for its antiseptic and antibacterial properties to aid in wound healing and soothe skin irritations.

5. **Potential for Diabetes Management:** Some studies suggest that curcumin might have benefits for individuals with diabetes. It may help in regulating blood sugar levels and improving insulin sensitivity, potentially aiding in diabetes management.

6. **Joint Health:** Turmeric's anti-inflammatory properties may be beneficial for joint health. It's been used traditionally to alleviate symptoms of osteoarthritis and rheumatoid arthritis, potentially reducing joint pain and stiffness.

7. **Gastrointestinal Support:** Turmeric's ability to stimulate bile production might aid in promoting a healthy digestive system by supporting the breakdown of fats and potentially reducing symptoms of indigestion or bloating.

8. **Liver Health:** Curcumin may have hepatoprotective properties, potentially supporting liver health by protecting liver cells from damage caused by toxins and oxidative stress.

9. **Skin Health:** Some people use turmeric topically for its potential benefits in improving skin conditions. Its anti-inflammatory and antimicrobial properties might help in managing acne, eczema, and other skin issues.

10. **Potential for Weight Management:** Some research suggests that curcumin might play a role in weight management by potentially reducing inflammation associated with obesity and aiding in metabolic processes, though more studies are needed.

11. **Antiviral and Antibacterial Properties:** Turmeric contains compounds that have demonstrated antiviral and antibacterial effects in laboratory studies, suggesting potential benefits in fighting infections.

While turmeric offers these potential health benefits, it's important to remember that using it as a supplement or for medicinal purposes should be done under guidance, especially if you have specific health conditions or are taking medications. Incorporating turmeric into a balanced diet is generally safe, but consuming excessively high amounts may cause adverse effects in some individuals. Consulting a healthcare professional is advised for personalized guidance.

VALERIAN

Valerian (Valeriana officinalis) is an herb native to Europe and parts of Asia, known for its medicinal properties and historical use as a natural remedy for various conditions, particularly related to sleep and relaxation.

Key features and uses of valerian:

- **Appearance:** Valerian is a flowering plant with clusters of small, sweet-smelling pink or white flowers. Its roots are the primary part used for medicinal purposes.

- **Medicinal Properties:** Valerian root contains compounds such as valerenic acid and various antioxidants, which are believed to contribute to its potential health benefits.

- **Attention and Focus:** In some instances, valerian has been used to improve concentration and focus, particularly in individuals experiencing stress-related focus issues.

- **Mood Enhancement:** Valerian might have mild mood-enhancing effects. Some individuals use it to achieve a sense of calmness and relaxation.

HEALTH BENEFITS:

1. **Migraine Relief:** Valerian's muscle-relaxing properties may extend to its potential to ease tension headaches or migraines. Some individuals use it as a natural remedy to alleviate headache-related discomfort.

2. **Cardiovascular Support:** Valerian has been suggested to have potential benefits for cardiovascular health. It might help in reducing blood pressure due to its relaxing effects, though more research is needed to confirm these effects.

3. **Anticonvulsant Properties:** Some studies suggest that valerian may possess anticonvulsant properties, potentially helping in reducing the severity or frequency of seizures. However, further research is required in this area.

4. **Menopausal Symptom Relief:** Valerian has been used by some women to manage symptoms associated with menopause, such as hot flashes, mood swings, or sleep disturbances. It's believed to offer mild relief from these symptoms.

5. **Sleep Aid:** Valerian has been traditionally used as a natural remedy to promote relaxation and improve sleep quality. It's commonly used to alleviate insomnia and mild sleep disorders. The herb is available in various forms, including capsules, extracts, teas, and tinctures.

6. **Anxiety and Stress Relief:** Valerian root has been suggested to have anxiolytic (anti-anxiety) effects and may help reduce stress and nervous tension. Some individuals use it to ease symptoms of anxiety or restlessness.

7. **Relaxation and Muscle Relaxant:** Valerian's sedative properties may contribute to its ability to induce relaxation. It's been used to soothe muscle tension and ease discomfort caused by muscle spasms.

8. **Stress-Related Gastrointestinal Discomfort:** Valerian's calming effects might extend to alleviating stress-related gastrointestinal discomforts, such as mild stomach upset or nervous stomach.

9. **Potential Anti-inflammatory Effects:** Some studies suggest that valerian extracts may possess anti-inflammatory properties. These properties might contribute to reducing inflammation in certain conditions, although more research is needed to validate these effects.

10. **Pain Management:** Valerian might have mild analgesic properties. Some individuals use it to alleviate mild pain or discomfort, though its effectiveness for pain relief requires further scientific investigation.

As with any herbal supplement or remedy, it's important to consult with a healthcare professional before using valerian, especially if you have specific health concerns, are pregnant, nursing, or taking medications. Valerian supplements can interact with certain medications or conditions, and guidance from a healthcare provider is recommended for safe and appropriate usage.

VERVAIN

Vervain, scientifically known as Verbena officinalis, is a flowering plant in the Verbenaceae family. It's a perennial herb native to Europe and Asia but has spread to other parts of the world, including North America, where it's often considered a weed.

Key features and uses of vervain:

- **Appearance:** Vervain has slender, erect stems that bear small, delicate clusters of lilac to pale blue flowers. Its lance-shaped leaves are arranged oppositely along the stems.

- **Cultural Significance:** Vervain has a rich history in various cultures and has been associated with several beliefs and traditions. It's been used in ancient rituals, herbal medicine, and even folklore, believed to possess various mystical or healing properties.

- **Medicinal Uses:** Traditionally, vervain has been used in herbal medicine for its potential medicinal benefits. It was historically used to treat a range of ailments, including headaches, anxiety, insomnia, digestive issues, and as a mild sedative. It's believed to have properties that promote relaxation and alleviate stress.

- **Culinary Uses:** In some culinary traditions, vervain has been used as a flavoring agent in teas, liqueurs, or herbal infusions due to its slightly bitter taste and aromatic qualities.

- **Wildlife Attraction:** Vervain's nectar-rich flowers are attractive to pollinators like bees and butterflies, making it a beneficial plant for supporting local ecosystems.

1. **Respiratory Support:** Vervain has been historically used to support respiratory health. It was believed to have expectorant properties, helping to clear mucus and ease respiratory discomforts like coughs or congestion.

2. **Mood Enhancement:** Some traditional uses of vervain suggest its potential to uplift mood and alleviate symptoms of mild depression or low spirits. It was believed to have mild calming effects on the nervous system.

3. **Menstrual Support:** Vervain has been used traditionally to address menstrual issues. It was believed to have mild antispasmodic properties that might alleviate menstrual cramps or discomfort.

4. **Digestive Aid:** In herbal medicine, vervain was used to aid digestion. It was believed to stimulate the production of digestive juices, potentially assisting in the digestive process.

5. **Antioxidant Properties:** Vervain contains certain compounds with antioxidant properties. These antioxidants may help neutralize harmful free radicals in the body, potentially reducing oxidative stress.

6. **Oral Health:** Vervain was used in some cultures for its potential in oral health. It was believed to have mild antiseptic properties that might contribute to maintaining oral hygiene.

7. **Wound Healing:** Some historical uses of vervain involved its application to minor wounds or cuts. It was believed to have properties that promote wound healing.

It's important to note that much of the information about the medicinal uses of vervain comes from traditional practices and historical beliefs. Modern scientific research on its health benefits is limited, and its effectiveness and safety for various health conditions require further investigation. Consulting with a healthcare professional before using vervain for medicinal purposes is advisable, especially if you have specific health concerns or are taking medications.

WHITE WILLOW BARK

White willow bark refers to the bark obtained from the white willow tree, scientifically known as Salix alba. This tree is native to Europe and parts of Asia, and it has been traditionally used for medicinal purposes for centuries. Here are key features and characteristics of white willow bark:

1. **Botanical Characteristics:** Salix alba is a deciduous tree that can grow up to 30 meters in height. It has long, narrow leaves with a distinctive silvery-white underside, giving the tree its common name.

2. **Bark:** The bark of the white willow tree is where the medicinal properties are primarily found. The bark is grayish-brown and has a bitter taste.

3. **Active Compounds:** White willow bark contains several compounds, with salicin being the most notable. Salicin is a natural precursor to salicylic acid, which is similar to the active ingredient in aspirin.

4. **Traditional Uses:** White willow bark has a long history of use in traditional medicine, dating back to ancient times. It has been used for its analgesic (pain-relieving), anti-inflammatory, and antipyretic (fever-reducing) properties.

HEALTH BENEFITS

1. **Pain Relief:** Due to its salicin content, white willow bark has been used as a natural remedy for pain relief, including headaches, muscle aches, and joint pain.

2. **Anti-Inflammatory Properties:** The anti-inflammatory properties of white willow bark may help reduce inflammation, making it potentially beneficial for conditions such as arthritis and other inflammatory disorders.

3. **Fever Reduction:** White willow bark has historically been used to lower fever, a use that aligns with its traditional role as an antipyretic agent.

4. **Aspirin Connection:** The development of aspirin is closely linked to the compounds found in white willow bark. Aspirin, a widely used pain reliever, was initially derived from salicin.

5. **Cautions and Considerations:** While white willow bark has been used as a natural alternative to aspirin, it is important to note that it can still have side effects, especially in higher doses. Individuals with certain medical conditions or those taking medications should consult with a healthcare professional before using white willow bark.

6. **Salicylate Sensitivity:** People with a known sensitivity to salicylates, such as those found in aspirin, should avoid using white willow bark or consult with a healthcare provider before doing so.

As with any herbal remedy, it's advisable to seek guidance from a healthcare professional before using white willow bark, especially if you have existing health conditions, are pregnant, or are taking other medications. Additionally, considering the potential side effects and interactions, it's crucial to use it in moderation and under appropriate supervision.

WORMWOOD

Wormwood, scientifically known as Artemisia absinthium, is an herbaceous perennial plant belonging to the Asteraceae family. It's native to Europe, Asia, and North Africa and is recognized for its bitter taste and potent aromatic properties.

Key features and uses of wormwood:

- **Appearance:** Wormwood has silvery-green, deeply lobed leaves that are covered in fine hairs. It produces small yellow flowers in clusters, typically during the summer.

- **Cultural Significance:** Wormwood has a long history of use dating back centuries, especially in herbal medicine and traditional practices. It gained notoriety as a key ingredient in the spirit absinthe, known for its bitter taste and distinctive green color.

- **Medicinal Uses:** In herbal medicine, wormwood was traditionally used for various purposes. It was believed to have anthelmintic properties, potentially helping in expelling intestinal parasites. It was also used to aid digestion, stimulate appetite, and relieve mild stomach discomfort.

- **Culinary Uses:** Despite its bitter taste, wormwood has occasionally been used as a flavoring agent in alcoholic beverages, particularly in historical preparations of absinthe. Its strong flavor meant it was used sparingly.

- **Caution:** Wormwood contains compounds like thujone, which in high concentrations, can be toxic and cause adverse effects such as seizures or organ damage. Due to its potential toxicity, it should be used cautiously, if at all, and only under professional guidance.

- **Insect Repellent:** Wormwood has been used as a natural insect repellent. Some cultures would place dried wormwood in closets or beds to ward off insects.

- ❧ **Historical Uses:** Throughout history, wormwood was also used in cultural and religious rituals and as a component in herbal remedies to address various ailments, including fevers and menstrual irregularities.

HEALTH BENEFITS:

1. **Potential Antimicrobial Properties:** Wormwood contains compounds that have shown some antimicrobial activity in laboratory studies. It was believed to inhibit the growth of certain bacteria and fungi, suggesting potential applications in managing microbial infections, though more research is needed.

2. **Appetite Stimulation:** In traditional herbal medicine, wormwood was used to stimulate appetite. It was believed to have properties that could aid digestion and promote the secretion of digestive juices, potentially increasing hunger.

3. **Menstrual Support:** Wormwood was historically used to regulate menstrual cycles and alleviate menstrual discomfort. It was believed to have mild antispasmodic properties that might ease menstrual cramps or irregularities.

4. **Potential Anti-inflammatory Effects:** Some research indicates that compounds in wormwood may possess anti-inflammatory properties. These properties might help reduce inflammation associated with certain conditions, although more studies are necessary to confirm these effects.

5. **Digestive Support:** Wormwood was traditionally used to support digestive health. It was believed to have properties that could ease mild stomach discomfort and aid in digestion, potentially improving overall gastrointestinal function.

6. **Relief from Skin Conditions:** In some traditional practices, wormwood was used topically to address minor skin irritations, such as itching or insect bites, due to its potential antiseptic properties.

7. **Anti-Fungal**: Wormwood's name stems from its historical use in treating parasites, including helminths such as pinworms, roundworms, and tapeworms that cause severe gastrointestinal disease. Historically, wormwood had been considered a preferred remedy for intestinal worms, but it dropped out of favor due to severe side effects associated with the liquor absinthe.

Wormwood contains compounds that can be toxic in high doses, and its use should be approached cautiously and under the guidance of a qualified healthcare professional. Pregnant or nursing individuals and those with certain health conditions should avoid its use. Always consult with a healthcare provider before using wormwood or any herbal remedy.